PRIMITIVE PEOPLES WITHOUT SALT:

A PERSPECTIVE FOR INDUSTRIALIZED SOCIETIES

William J. Oliver, M.D.

Publisher's Cataloging-in-Publication
(Provided by Quality Books, Inc.)

Oliver, William John, 1925-
Primitive peoples without salt : a perspective for industrialized societies / William J. Oliver. -- 1st ed.

p. cm.
Includes bibliographical references and index.
Preassigned LCCN: 97-92346
ISBN: 0-9658325-0-3

1. Salt-free diet. 2. Salt in the body. 3. Salt--Physiological effect. 4. Yanomamo Indians--Nutrition. 5. Yanomamo Indians--Health and hygiene. I. Title.

RM237.8.O55 1998 613.2'85'0898
QBI98-30

To Marguerite, whose love, encouragement and support for over fifty years made this book and other accomplishments possible.

Contents

Preface

This book, as described in the introductory chapter, introduces the concept that healthy existence in a salt (sodium chloride) poor environment was the normal dietary pattern in many groups in the pre-Columbian period. My personal studies of one such group, the Yanomamö Amerindians, stimulated my interest in retrieving from the literature information on other groups flourishing in a similar salt poor state. In an attempt to understand the physiological responses permitting this successful existence, the human data have been put into evolutionary perspective in an extensive review of the phylogenetic emergence of adaptations to achieve sodium homeostasis.

The initial sequence of events leading to this book commenced some thirty years ago. At that time, Professor James V. Neel, the Chairman of the Department of Human Genetics of the University of Michigan, accepted me as a member of his multidisciplinary team to perform various biomedical studies on the isolated Yanomamö Amerindians living in the interior of Brazil and Venezuela among the headwaters of the Amazon and Orinoco Rivers. On first inspection, these primitive peoples displayed robust general health at all ages. On detailed observations of their diet, the Yanomamö were remarkable in representing a "no-salt" culture, having neither dietary sources of mineral sodium chloride nor substances of high salinity. For a pediatric nephrologist, these people represented a unique society for study of successful sodium homeostasis in an extremely salt poor environment. Professor Neel's philosophy of encouraging each member of the investigating team to initiate a research project among the Yanomamö permitted my studies of sodium balance and associated hormonal adjustments. Importantly, Dr. Neel's philosophy extended to the protocol that all members of the team assist one another in as much as feasible in the collection of data and samples, whether demographic characteristics, linguistic lists, anthropometric measurements, or samples of blood, urine and other biologic fluids. This assistance was critical to the success of my studies. The further imposition of serving as acculturated controls for

Preface

the native subjects extended my fellow investigators' investment in my research.

Communication with the Yanomamö in their unique language was essential to conducting what would appear to these isolated people to be, at best, weird in the collection of urine and fecal samples, and even more ludicrous in our payment in the form of knifes and machetes for their excreta. A twenty-four hour urine collection in a large plastic container was even more of a joke to these people. Dr. Napoleon A. Chagnon gave invaluable assistance in this critical task of explaining the research protocol to the Yanomamö on five of the six field studies during which my observations and collections were made. On one of the six expeditions, Dr. Earnesto Migliazza served as the linguist for my work. Their effectiveness in provision of the linguistic needs for my studies was fully reflected in the array of data I was able to collect in these unacculturated people.

With exception of Drs. Neel and Chagnon, the participants on the field trips conducted over a span of some twenty years (1967-1987) varied according the particular goals of the planned studies. Many members of the teams greatly assisted me in my data and sample collections. These included: Dr. Raymond Hames, Mrs. Priscilla Neel, Dr. Richard Spielman and Mrs. Karen Spielman. Other members of the expeditions played some part in my data collections but limitation of space does not permit a full listing of all participants.

The essential laboratory analyses required for my studies were conducted primarily by collaborators among the faculty of the University of Michigan. These were: Dr. Edwin L. Cohen, Dr. Warren C. Eveland and Dr. Robert Grekin. Dr. W. Nowaczynski of the University of British Columbia performed the measurements of aldosterone and protein-binding variables.

An appreciation of the paucity of sodium in the customary foods of the Yanomamö and the possible contributions to sodium intake associated with cooking practices and tobacco

Preface

use required precise analyses of representative samples. These analyses were generously performed in the Analytical Chemistry Laboratories of the Gerber Products Company of Fremont, Michgan under the supervision of Dr. George A. Purvis, Director of Nutrition, and Dr. Sandra Pfieffer, Group Leader of the Analytical Chemistry Division.

Professor Neel, in addition to his position as senior investigator for the multiple expeditions in which I was a member, has been an active participant in the interpretation of the collected data and in the writing of the final manuscripts for publication. His collaboration greatly enhanced appreciation of the significance of the findings and the clarity of presentation of the finished manuscripts.

My knowledge and understanding of other studies and publications describing previously identified isolated groups originally living in salt-free cultures have been greatly expanded by discussions with other investigators. These include, especially, the late Dr. Lot Page, Dr. Malcolm Holliday, and Dr. William Harlem.

I am deeply indebted to Dr. Derek Denton, Director Emeritus of the Howard Florey Institute of Experimental Physiology and Medicine of Melbourne, Australia for his generous sharing of his work on all aspects of salt appetite in nonprimate animals. During a several months' visiting professorship in early 1980, Dr. Denton and his colleagues provided me with their published and unpublished data and were unstinting in allocating unrestrained time for discussion for my edification on salt appetite in comparative animals. In addition to Dr. Denton, these scientists included: Dr. John Blair-West, Dr. John Coghlan, Dr. Marelyn Wintour-Coghlan, and Dr. Bruce Scoggins. The cordiality that these investigators and their families extended to my wife and me socially added a further positive diminsion to our time in Australia.

December 1997
Ann Arbor, Michigan

Acknowledgements

For tables reproduced in this book from other publications, beneath each is an acknowledgement of the authors. The bibliographic source is included in the references for the chapter in which these appear. In each instance, permission was also obtained for reproduction. All other tables represent previously published data by the author with the appropriate source or unpublished data of the author.

Figure III-1 was reproduced by permission of Holt, Rinehart and Winston. Figure III-6 was kindly provided by Dr. Earnesto Migliazza. Figure X-1 was reproduced with permission of the Journal of the American Medical Association. All other figures represent original material developed by the author or photographs taken by the author.

Financial support for the research performed by the author and described in this book has been provided by multiple sources. These are appropriately acknowledged in the original publications detailing my studies of the Yanomamö and Guaymi Amerindians.

Primitive Peoples Without Salt

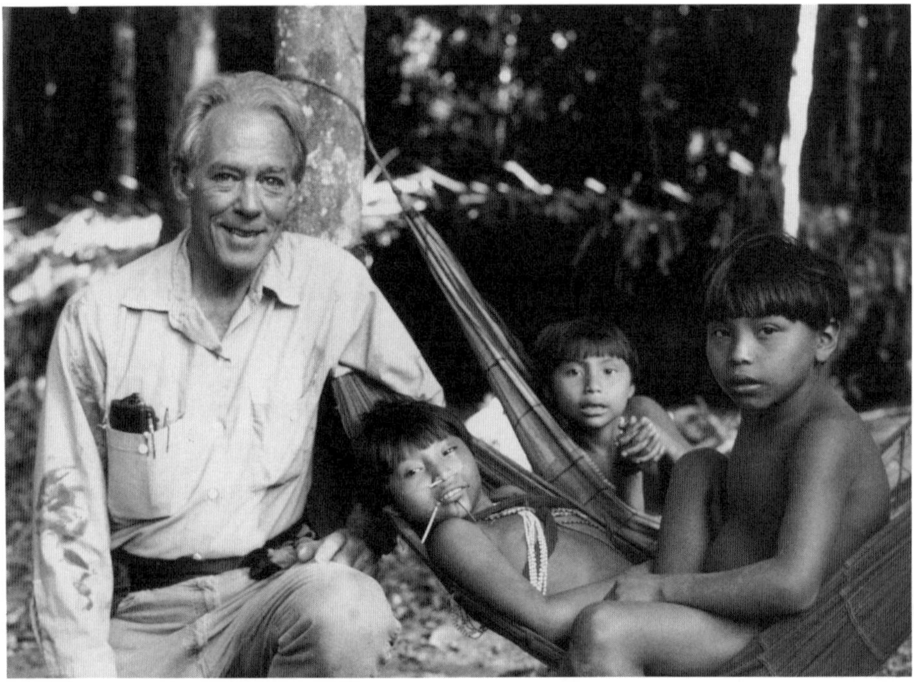

The author with Yanomamö Amerindian children.

I. Introduction

Survival and health of man in the absence of mineral salt (sodium chloride) or substances of high salinity in the diet have been observed in unacculturated peoples (Alpers, 1965; Holmberg, 1950; Kroeber, 1941-42; Morse, 1937; Oliver, 1975; Stefansson, 1922). Perusal of these publications documents a wide geographic distribution of these "salt-free" cultures. Among them there are major differences in racial and ethnic groups, local climates, tribal customs, dietary patterns, and modes of subsistence. Subsequent discussions of these observations by others often imply a pathological uniqueness of the ethnic group under consideration when contrasted with dietary characteristics of the vast industrialized populations of the world (Dawber, 1967; Pickering, 1981). A diametrically counter view is the concept that "salt-free" cultures represent the true normal pattern of dietary subsistence of man (Dahl, 1958; Meneely, 1961). The fact of the matter is that salt-free cultures prevailed in a large portion of the native populations initially contacted in the post-Columbian era. Not a universality, but as will be described, many of the peoples inhabiting the American continents, Africa, Australia, Oceania, and several other geographic sites existed without salt in the pre-Columbian period. The data substantiating the existence of this dietary state will be reviewed for various ethnic groups including those previously reported to be salt-free cultures plus others not previously recognized to have existed in a no-salt culture prior to civilized contact.

Before reviewing observations consistent with the concept that subsistence upon a no-salt diet is indeed the normal physiological state for man, a brief consideration of the chronology of contact and commerce in various parts of the early civilized societies of North Africa, Asia, and Europe can provide a useful background and, perhaps, a perspective for explaining the almost universal use of salt as a condiment and as a preservative by nearly all acculturated groups. Commencing before 3,000 years B.C., the first civilizations evolved in several sites including Crete, Mesopotamia, and Egypt; they are believed to have developed in that sequence. Within the eastern portion of the Mediterranean Sea, the Cretans established one of the earliest intercontinental trade routes to North Africa, Asia Minor, and the shores of the Near East. Over the next 2,400 years, new civilizations rose while old ones were destroyed by external forces or internal rebellion. Throughout this interval, contacts between peoples by peaceful trade and commerce or by military incursion occurred repeatedly and intensely across Asia, Europe, and North Africa. These exchanges resulted in the introduction and adoption of cross-culture customs, ideas, and technologies. Certain of these, such as use of the wheel, domestication of animals, and techniques of agriculture became almost universal throughout these vast geographic areas constituting the known world of the second millennium A.D. Older literature of Arabic, Greek, Jewish, and Persian origin and the location of ancient mines and their associated trade routes for the mineral suggest that use of salt was also a common cross-cultural custom (Benton, 1973). The common usage of salt in the recorded history of man is well substantiated by the presence of over 30 references to the mineral as a condiment and as a preservative for meat in both the old and the new testaments of the Bible (Hartman, 1963).

In contrast to the intense degree of contact between the various civilized societies of Asia, Europe, and North Africa during the period of recorded history, albeit over many millennia, the inhabitants of the then undiscovered and unexplored regions represented by the interior of Africa, the continents of the Americas, Australia, and Oceania (the islands of the Pacific, including New Zealand) engaged in trade but were limited in cross-cultural contacts. This restriction resulted from the relative geographic isolation consequent to dense jungle terrain or oceans and seas of varying dimensions. These isolated areas were populated with various racial and ethnic groups represented by aborigines, Amerindians, Melanesians, Micronesians, Negroes, Polynesians, and others.

Other background facts are important from the perspective of a review of no-salt cultures. The initial contact with various primitive groups has occurred at differing times throughout the post-Columbian era, including even the past two decades (Nance, 1975). The backgrounds of those making first contact with unacculturated groups are highly diverse, ranging from early explorers, itinerant traders, and proselyting missionaries to scientists trained in a spectrum of disciplines and supported by a wealth of sophisticated equipment and laboratory capabilities. Obviously, the quality of information resulting from observations during initial contacts will extend, hopefully, from accurate and adequate descriptive recordings to thoughtfully planned collections and analyses of biological samples and major dietary staples accompanied by comprehensive observations on important associated environmental and other phenomena. Inclusion in the available contemporary studies of data related to the hormonal adjustments coincident to a sodium-sparse environment provides a dimension to understanding the physiological adaptations occasioned by a lifetime on a salt-poor diet.

For even the best of attempts, data obtained during field expeditions to isolated groups can never achieve the precision to be achieved in a classical metabolic study in a hospital setting. Nevertheless, from our experience with the Yanomamö Indians (Oliver, 1975; Oliver, 1981) and those recorded by other investigators, the observation that the group in question does not use salt or substances of high salinity can be substantiated by chemical analyses on aliquots of 24 hour urine collections. That such analyses accurately reflect intake of sodium chloride at either high or low levels has been previously documented (Dahl, 1958; Meneely, 1961). These combinations of field observations describing a no-salt culture substantiated by chemical analyses of timed urine collections have an additional implication. They provide some credence for validating the detailed observations by various recorders who have differing backgrounds and disciplines and who have described other no-salt cultures at the time of initial or early contact by non-natives, but without data on urinary sodium excretion. The validity of such observations is enhanced when reports by several independent observers exist. The conclusion from the observation that a particular ethnic group is not using salt does not require a scientific background; rather, a keen observer who is also a meticulous recorder. Thus, the detailed recordings of explorers, traders, missionaries, anthropologists, and others may provide data pertinent to the dietary pattern of a particular people. From this perspective, the extent of salt-free cultures existing prior to acculturated contact can be considerably increased. This possibility will be examined for various groups who were initially recognized in the post-Columbian era.

It is pertinent to recall that an appetite for salt by man is easily and rapidly acquired. This observation has been exploited over the years by various individuals and organizations, for example, traders and missionaries, for the barter of native goods or to gain the proximity of the primitive for instruction in religion and other subjects (Chagnon, 1980; Helm, 1979; Holmberg, 1950). Given the pragmatic fact that salt is a cheap commodity as a consequence of commercial production and one that is easily transported, it is obviously a practical choice as a trade item. As a consequence of the general belief that salt is a requirement in the diet for health, an additional advantage seemingly accrues from the intruder providing the mineral to newly contacted groups. Foods preserved in salt, such as tinned meat, serve as a further source of sodium in the diet. We have observed this pattern in some Yanomamö Indians to the extent that in certain villages with established government or missionary posts the observed intake of salt and measured excretion of sodium in the urine approach levels found in our usual acculturated societies of today. This departure from a culture that existed for at least several thousands years without salt to one quite satiated with the mineral has occurred in only 30 years in some Yanomamö villages! The observation also emphasizes the fact that the true dietary state of a primitive group regarding sodium intake can be rapidly obliterated by a relatively short time of acculturated contact. This phenomenon has been noted by several observers (Chagnon, 1980; Helm, 1979; Holmberg, 1950). Thus, the actual native diet of a group under consideration requires observations at the time of first contact or within a brief interval prior to establishment of even the most limited trade exchanges with acculturated groups.

There are two additional approaches by which salt-free cultures can be identified. The first is the determination that the group in question had no word in their original language for salt or salty substances. However, since languages are constantly changing, it is essential to distinguish between words which were originally in the language versus those added or devised after initial acculturated contact.

The second approach is the use of the culture element distribution list from which the identified informant is asked whether a particular item was used within the native culture (Kroeber, 1941-42). The list includes questions on whether the group hunted certain specific animals, used or excluded certain animals from the diet, and used or did not use specific techniques in food preparation and storage. This technique has been extensively used in anthropological studies of Amerindians of the western portion of North America.

Primitive Peoples Without Salt

If, in the course of examination of the available information, a particular tribal or ethnic group of peoples can be identified to have lived in a no-salt culture, it is not necessary that all the related peoples of that geographic area live on a no-salt diet. For the group under consideration, it is logical to believe that all individuals constituting the group possess those necessary adaptive physiological processes to maintain sodium homeostasis in the absence of dietary salt. In relation to sodium homeostasis, it is even more reassuring if, by observation or by pattern of migration, data supporting an expansion of the race or ethnic group can be documented. Such expansion substantiates the absence of a selective disadvantage conferred by existence on a salt-free diet.

For purposes of organization, the presentation will follow in general the geographic regions in respect to post-Columbian contact. This will permit an orderly consideration of the descriptions and data regarding the various peoples.

Introduction

II. North America

Simultaneously with the discovery of America in 1492 by Columbus, Bretons, Normans, and Englishmen in a search for new fishing grounds had sailed to the shores of Labrador and Newfoundland into the gulf of the St. Lawrence River and further south in proximity to Cape Cod (Terrell, 1971). During the subsequent four centuries, exploration by Europeans of many nationalities resulted in the contact of nearly all groups and tribes of Amerindians and Eskimos in North America. Permeation of the native custom and diet with acculturated goods and practices effectively obliterated any opportunity of obtaining valid measurements of urinary sodium excretion of North Amerindians ingesting a native pre-Columbian diet. Thus, information of the pre-Columbian diet of North Amerindians and Eskimos cannot include estimates of sodium intake by diet analyses or measurements of the urinary excretion of that element but are limited to observational reports with one exception for Eskimos (Rabinowitch, 1937).

A further complication exists in consideration of pre-Columbian dietary patterns in in North America. Although not a consistent problem, some of the reputed early accounts of dietary patterns of North Amerindians are in fact the first reports by English-speaking observers who established contact following earlier encounters by French and Spanish explorers. For example, the technique of hardening salt by exposure to fire was allegedly taught to coastal Indians by the Spanish (Eskew, 1948). Thus, as noted in the introduction, valid observations and reports of dietary characteristics are limited to those made upon initial or extremely early contact. Some, however, appear to be quite explicit. Among the informative sources is *A Memoir of Jacques Cartier*, translated by Baxter (1906). Cartier, one of the early French explorers of North America, made three voyages to the North American continent and explored the St. Lawrence River and its tributaries westward to the site of the present-day

Montreal. In 1535 on his second voyage, Cartier vividly described the dietary practices of the Wyandot Indians whom the French called Hurons. In describing the Indian village named Hochelaga, at the site of Montreal, Cartier commented:

"There are within this town about fifty long houses of about fifty paces or more each, and twelve or fifteen paces wide, and all made of timbers covered and garnished with great pieces of bark and strips of the said timber, as broad as tables, well tied artificially according to their manner. And within these there are many lodgings and chambers, and in the middle of these houses there is a great room on the ground where they make their fire and live in common; after that the men retire with their wives and children to their said chambers. Likewise they have granaries at the top of their houses where they put their corn of which they make their bread, which they call *carraconny*, and they make it in the manner following: they have mortars of wood as for braying flax, and beat the said corn into powder with pestles of wood; then they mix it into paste and make round cakes of it, which they put on a broad stone that is hot; then they cover it with hot stones, and so bake their bread instead of in an oven. They make likewise many stews of the said corn, and beans and peas, of which they have enough, and also of big cucumbers and other fruits. They have also in their houses great vessels like tuns, where they put their fish, namely eels and others, which they dry in the smoke during the summer and live upon it in the winter. And of this they make a great store, as we have seen by experience. All their living is without any taste of salt, and they lie on barks of trees stretched upon the earth, with wretched coverings of skins from which they make their clothing - namely wolves, beavers, martens, foxes, wild cats, deer, stags, and other wild beasts; but the most part of them go almost entirely naked."

During the time spent in Hochelaga by Cartier and his men, the following account was given:

"Then our said captain took a prayer-book and read full loudly, word by word, the passion of our Lord, so that all the bystanders could hear it, while all these poor people kept a great silence and were marvelously good hearers, looking up to heaven and making the same ceremonies that they saw us make; after which the captain made all the men range themselves on one side, the women on another and the children another, and gave to the chiefs hatchets, to the others knives, and to the women paternosters and other trifling articles; then he threw into the midst of the place among the little children some small rings and Agnus Dei of tin, at which they showed a marvelous joy. This done, the said captain commanded the trumpets and other instruments of music to sound, with which the said people were greatly delighted; after which things we took leave of them and withdrew. Seeing this, the women put themselves before us to stop us, and brought us of their victuals, which they had prepared for us, as fish, stews, beans, and other things, thinking to make us eat and dine at the said place; and because their victuals were not to our taste and had no savor of salt, we thanked them, making them a sign that we did not need to eat."

In comments prefacing Cartier's account of his impressions of the Hochelagan village, Baxter noted: "In 'great vessels like tuns' was kept the fish which had been smoked during the summer for winter's use. Like many other Indian tribes of North America, the Hochelagans used no salt whatever in their food, which comprised game and fish, maize, beans, peas, pumpkins, cucumbers, and wild fruits."

Among the additional explorations translated by Baxter (1906) is "The Voyage of John Francis de la Rocque, Knights, Lord of Roberval," who also explored the St. Lawrence River up to the site of present-day Montreal in 1542. In a discussion entitled "The Manners of the Savages," de la Rocque provided the following description:

"Instead of apparel they wear skins upon them like mantles, and they have a small pair of breeches, where with they cover their privities, as well men as women. They have hosen and shoes of leather, excellently made; and they have no shirts, neither cover they their heads; but their hair is trussed up above the crown of their heads and plaited or braided. Touching their victuals, they eat good meat, but all unsalted, but they dry it, and afterward they broil it, as well fish as flesh. They have no certain dwelling-place, and they go from place to place, as they think they may best find food, as aloses in one place, and other fish, salmons, sturgeons, mullets, surmullets, bass, carps, eels, pinperneaux and other fresh-water fish, and store of porpoises. They feed also of stags, wild boars, bugles, porkespines, and store of other wild beasts; and there is as great store of fowls as they can desire.

"Touching their bread, they make very good, and it is of great mill; and they live very well, for they take care for nothing else."

A subsequent account of the dietary habits of the Indians in the vicinity of the St. Lawrence River near the present site of Quebec was given by Joseph Jouvency, a priest and historian of the Society of Jesus. In 1710 in a monograph, "Concerning the Country and Manners of the Canadians, or the Savages of New France," Jouvency specifically referred to several of the Indian tribes who inhabited the northeastern woodlands and who were served by his brother missionaries during the period commencing in the year 1610. Among the tribes in the earlier portion of his discussion of their manners and customs, he included the Hurons, the Iroquois, the Montagnais, the Neutrals, and the Tobacco nation. Subsequently, he described their dietary habits.

North America

"Neither table nor chair can be seen in the hut. They squat upon their haunches like monkeys; this is their custom while eating, deliberating or conversing. They greet approaching friends with silly laughter, more often exclaiming, 'ho, hho, hhho.' When they eat they do not take beverages with their food, nor do they drink often, but only once after eating. Whoever entertains his friends at a feast neither sits with them nor touches any part of the food, but divides it among the feasters; or, if he has someone act as carver, sits apart fasting and looks on. While eating they keep silent; they reject salt and condiments; they consider it a sin to throw the bones to the dogs; they either burn them in the fire or bury them in the ground, for, they say, 'If the bears, beaver, and other wild animals which we capture in hunting should know that their bones were given to dogs and broken to pieces, they would not suffer themselves to be taken so easily.' They wipe off upon their hair the grease which has collected from fatty foods; some times they smear their cheeks or arms for the sake, as they say, of elegance and health; for they think that not only is the skin made resplendent with grease, but the limbs are strengthened."

Geographic locations of these tribes were in the general vicinity of the upper reaches of the St. Lawrence River and north and south of Lake Erie and Lake Ontario. In consideration of the possible extent of the Northeastern Indian tribes to be characteristically members of a no-salt culture, it is pertinent to consider a second article by Jouvency appearing in the same volume. Within that article, he provides a specific description of the names and geographic locations of the more than 30 missions of the Society of Jesus that existed in 1703. These extend from a northern site on the Saguenay River flowing southward into the midpoint of the St. Lawrence River to a more southerly route through Montreal then northwestward to the site of present-day Sault Ste. Marie, Michigan, then southwestward through the junction of the Des Plaines River and Kankakee River southwest of Lake Michigan in the present state of Illinois. Inasmuch as Jouvency points out differing customs observed in certain of the tribes, but provides only a single description of the general characteristics of the mealtime habits, as well as the preparation of food, it can be speculated that at the time of initial or early contact the many different tribes inhabiting the geographic areas in which the various individual missionary stations were located could be uniformly described as no-salt cultures. This speculation is potentially further supported by the earlier observations described previously. The various Indian tribes occupying these geographic areas included the Algonquions, the Montagnaises, the Abnakis, the Iroquois, the Illinois, the Eries, the Miamis, the Ottawas, the Potawatomis, the Neutrals, and the Tionontatis.

The methods for preservation of food used by the Illinois Indians living in the proximity of the junction of the Fox and Des Plaines River in the present-day state of Illinois were described by Pierre Liette, a French officer who lived with them for an extended period (Quaife, 1947). He described a buffalo hunt in 1688 and the technique employed in preserving the obtained meat for future use:

"To return to the hunt in which our savages engaged, they killed 120 buffaloes, from which they brought back a hundred tongues. The people from my cabin smoked these and destributed them among themselves to carry to me.

"We remained a week in this place in order to dry all this meat. For this purpose they make a kind of cradle ten feet long, three feet wide, and four feet high, which they call *gris*, upon which they spread out their meat after preparing it. Under this they kindle a little fire. It usually takes them a day to dry a flat side. There are two of these in a buffalo. They take it from the shoulder clear to the thigh and from the hump to the middle of the belly, after which they spread it out as thin as they can, usually making it four feet square. They fold it up while still hot, like a portfolio, so as to make it easier to carry. The strongest men and women carry as many as eight for the whole day. This is not possible in autumn nor in winter, however, as the cows are then very fat; they can then carry four at most."

He subsequently described the methods employed for preserving corn, pumpkins, several root crops, and wild onions:

"To return to the occupations of the women, at the end of July they begin to mix or dry the corn. They make two kinds. That which they roast gives them more trouble than that which they boil, for they have to make large griddles and take particular care to turn the ears from time to time to prevent their burning too much on one side, and afterwards they have to shell off the kernels. They therefore make very little of this kind. The kind which they boil they gather just as tender as the corn for roasting, and with shells, which they find more convenient than knives, they cut off all the kernels, throwing away the cobs, until they have as much as they wish to cook for that day. They never keep any for the next day because of the excessive care required to prevent it from turning sour. After it has boiled for a few minutes they spread it on reed mats, which they make in the same manner as those that serve for their cabins. The drying process usually takes two days. They make a great store of food of this kind.

"They have an abundant supply of fine pumpkins. They have a way of drying them that is not common to all the nations of this region, by which they keep from one year to the next. They scrape the rind well, and take out all the inside, and cut them into circular slices an inch thick. They let them dry for a day in the air, after which they tie them up, putting as many as five pumpkins together in this way. Then they expose them to the sun for several days, which dries them out so thoroughly that they break like a turnip. They cook this with meat and corn. It is a great treat among them. The French always make a liberal stock of this food.

"There are also many roots which the women gather. The one which they like best is the *macopine.* This is a big root which they get in the marshes. I have never tried to learn what the flower is like, so I cannot describe it, although I have seen the women pull the roots up from the ground at the bottom of the water, into which they sometimes wade up to the waist, and often duck their heads under the water to pluck them up. Some of them are as big as one's leg. The savages say that they are poisonous when raw, which I hardly believe.

"The women have unusual difficulty in cooking them. Sometimes three or four cabins combine and dig a hole in the ground five or six feet deep and ten or twelve square. They throw a lot of wood into it, which they set on fire, and when it is burning briskly they throw in a number of stones which they turn over with big levers until they are red hot. Then they go in quest of a large quantity of grass which they get at the bottom of the water and which they spread over the stones as well as they can to the thickness of about a foot. After this they throw in many buckets of water, and then each cabin puts its roots in its own place as fast as they can, covering them over with dry grass and bark and finally earth. They leave them thus for three days, during which they shrink to half their former size.

"In these same marshes they also gather other roots which are big as one's arm and all full of holes. These give them no trouble to prepare; they merely cut them into pieces half as thick as one's wrist, string them, and hang them in the sun or in the smoke to dry. This root has large leaves that spread out on the water, like the plant we call votets, but they are much larger. Between two of these leaves grows an object shaped like the body of a drinking-glass in which are the seeds, which are as big as hazelnuts. They also store up onions as big as Jerusalem artichokes, which they find in the prairies, and which I think are better than all the other roots. They are sugary and pleasing to the palate. They are cooked like the *macopines*."

Liette also provided an interesting description of the preparation and cooking of food while on a hunting expedition.

"When I came for the broiled meat on which they had promised to feast me, I could not understand where they would get means for cooking it. They took a fillet from within the body, this being the most tender part of all sorts of animals, and cut it into strips like sausages. One of them went off three or four *arpents* (French measurement approximating 193 feet) into a hollow, which in spring is nothing but a sort of marsh, and brought back a bundle of round reeds as thick as one's fingers. They drew from their quivers two bits of wood which serve them for striking a flame, and in almost no time they had a fire. They kindled a part of their reeds, over which they put their meat, which they turned from time to time with their bows. In spite of all the care they took to scrape it with their knives some ash remained, which rendered it as black as itself. Nevertheless, I ate heartily and found it very good. It was very tender and I had a good appetite."

Of interest is the description of cannibalism practiced by the Illinois Indians also given by Liette. During the time Liette spent living with the Illinois Indians, he had the opportunity to observe firsthand the behavior of these Indians regarding prisoners captured in a war or raid:

"When he (the captured warrior) is condemned to die, it is always by fire. I have never seen any other kind of torment used by this nation. They plant a little tree in the earth, which they make him clasp; they tie his wrists, and burn him with torches of straw or firebrands, sometimes for six hours. When they find his strength is almost spent they unfasten him and cut his thumbs off, after which they let him, if he wishes, run after those who are throwing stones at him, or who are trying to burn him. They even give him sticks which he holds with great difficulty. If he tries to run after anybody, they push him and he falls on his face, at which they hoot. Sometimes he furnishes a whole hour of diversion to these barbarians.

"Finally he succumbs under the strain of his torments, and sometimes drops down motionless. The rabble run to get firebrands, which they poke into the most sensitive parts of his body; they dray him over hot embers, which brings him back to life, at which they renew their hooting, as if theyhad performed some fine exploit. When they are tired of their sport, an old scoundrel cuts his flesh from the top of the nose to the chin and leaves it hanging, which gives him a horrible appearance. In this state they play a thousand tricks on him, and finally stone him or disembowel him. Some drink drink his blood. Women bring their male children still at the breast and place their feet in his body and wash them with his blood. They eat his heart raw.

"There are men and women who might be called cannibals, and who are called maneaters because they never fail to eat all of those who are put to death in their villages. At nightfall everybody, big and little, knocks loudly with big sticks on the cabins and on their scaffolds in order, as they say, to drive away from their village the soul of the man they have killed."

As noted by Quaife, Editor of the Memoirs of Leitte, cannibalism was practised by many tribes of North American Indians. It has been suggested that the practice was more symbolic in that the admirable qualities of the slain individual would be transferred to those indulging in cannibalism. Quaife commented that additional accounts of cannibalism include the victorious Indians at the Mackinaw Massacre of 1763 feasting upon the body of one of the slaughtered Englishmen, and the Indians at the Chicago Massacre of August 15, 1812 eating the heart of Captain William Wells.

Interesting observations were recorded by Oliver M. Spencer who was a captive of the Mohawk Indians who at that time occupied land in northern Ohio near the site of the confluence of the Auglaize and Maumee Rivers (Quaife, 1917). Spencer was born in 1780 and was captured by a raiding party of Mohawks in July of 1792 and remained a captive until the end of February 1793, when his freedom was purchased by a British agent. In describing his travels from the site of capture slightly north of Cincinnati, Spencer commented:

"We encamped this evening about sunset in a low rich bottom near a beautiful stream; where having made a fire and roasted part of a young fawn which White Loon (one of the two Indians) a few minutes before had killed, we ate a very hearty supper, though without salt or bread...."

Subsequently, he described another meal with his Indian captors, again during the course of his travels to their native village:

"In the course of a few hours traveling this morning, crossing a great many small branches running in various directions and then passing through a very extensive prairie, we came to a stream running northwardly, and following its course until noon halted by the side of a small rivulet. Having no provisions Wawpawmawquaw went to hunt some, but soon returned unsuccessful. Just at this time a large hawk flying over our heads with a snake in its talons and alighting on a tree a short distance from us was brought down with a rifle, and being dressed by plucking out the larger and singeing off the smaller feathers, and then boiled in our brass kettle with a quantity of milkweed, in about half an hour furnished us a dinner of flesh, soup, and greens. Even the Indians ate sparingly; for myself, though hungry, I found the hawk so touch and strong that I could eat but a few mouthfuls; as for the soup and greens, without salt the taste was not only insipid, but sickening."

At the time of the initial European contact by the Spanish, the Muskogee, who are better known as the Creek Indians, were located geographically along the Atlantic coast of Georgia to the vicinity of the Savannah River and westerly through central Alabama to the eastern border of the present-day state of Mississippi. As noted by Terrell (1971), the Muskogees united a nucleus of other tribes into a much larger cooperative group which ultimately became known as the Creek Confederacy. The amalgamated tribes included the Apalachicola, Hitchiti, Okmulgee, Sawokli, Chiaha, Asochi, Yuchi, Alabama, Tawasa, Pawotke, Muklasa, Koasati, Tuskegee, and sections of the Shawnee, Guale, and Yimasee tribes. Although Terrell considers that no reasonable estimate of the population of the Creek Confederacy at its height are available, it is estimated that there may have been an excess of 300 Creek villages at the zenith of the Confederacy.

One of the most comprehensive observers of Creek life and customs was Colonel Benjamin Hawkins, the United States Agent for Indian Affairs for all of the area south of the Ohio River for the period from 1796 to 1806. His observations comprise nine volumes written by Hawkins himself, plus one written by his secretary, Richard Thomas. In his appointment as agent for Indian affairs, he deserted the North Carolina of his origin and devoted himself entirely to the Indians of his assigned territory. From his established Indian agency on the Flint River in the area of Crawford County, Georgia, Hawkins traveled widely throughout the Creek Confederacy. In his account (1848) entitled "A Sketch of the Creek Country in the Years 1796-1799," he described general customs and dietary characteristics of the Creek tribe:

"I sat out at nine down the creek and in half a mile crossed Aquonausete running to the right 75 feet wide. Since I left the mountains yesterday, I find that I am on the Creek waters. This river is the Tallapoosa.

"I encamped on a creek margined with cane, running to the right. All these waters empty into Aquonausete. My guide in the evening told me we had traveled 34 miles -- here I saw a Creek Indian, near his hunting camp, he at first was a great distance from me and walked hastily on till he came up with me, gave me his hand, told me who he was and conversed for some time with my guide, who had been instructed to inform everyone who he saw in the path who I was. In the course of the evening it rained. I had prepared for a shelter in time which was covered with a blanket, bear skins and oilcloth cloak. I was surprised at the little effect the rain had on my two Indians, the old man had a leather shirt and legings, the younger one leather legings and an old shirt, they had each a small halfworn blanket, the young man every evening pulled off his shirt and spread it under him. They both slept soundly the whole time it rained, got up once and ordered my attendants up twice to endeavor to preserve our fire by the addition of wood, but they never stirred till daybreak; they are small eaters, use no salt, and but little bread. They carried their parched cornmeal, *wissoetaw*, and mixed a handful in a pint of water which they drink. Although they had plenty of corn and fowls, they made no other provision than a small bag of this for the path . . . I have several times drank of the *wissoetaw* and am fond of it with the addition of some sugar. To make of the best quality I am told the corn should be first boiled, then parched in hot ashes, sifted, pounded and made into flour."

Additional observations by Hawkins concern the introduction to the Creek Indians of salt for the preservation of meat:

"The women immediately brought some fowls which were very fat, and made the necessary provisions for me here and for the road. They asked a pint of salt a pair for fat hens, and a quart for a bushel of corn. I had a long conversation with them on the situation and circumstances as it respected their labor and required to know what they made and what they wished, in aid of their own exertions. They informed me they performed almost all the labor, the men assisted but little and that in the corn. They generally made a plenty of corn and sweet potatoes and pumpkins. They made beans, corn peas, cymblins, gourds, watermelons, muskmelons, collards and onions. They made great use of beans in their bread.

"They wanted principally salt, that they used but little from necessity, and where they were able to supply themselves plentifully with meat, they were unable to preserve it for the want of salt. They raised hogs, some cattle, and a great many poultry."

At the entrance of the little Chota Creek into the Chattahoochee River, Hawkins described the conditions of a small tribe of Creek Indians in the village of Looccunna:

"I was here informed of some of the difficulties and hardships which these poor people are subject to. They sell the fowls grown, two for 21/2 yards of binding worth 2 cents, a bushel of corn for a quart of salt and sometimes a pint, and the woman had just returned from the settlements, a journey of 17 days."

North America

The prominence of trade in salt is vividly pictured in one profile by Hawkins detailing the return of Creek Indians of the Chattahoochee River region from a trading post:

"Some Indians of the Cusseta returning from St. Mary's informed me that they had suffered much on the path with hunger, there being no game of any kind to be had and provisions were scarce there . . . . They called to see me, to talk with me, and as it was their duty, to inform me that some of those who were down did not conduct themselves as well as they ought to have done, that they had killed some beef, and that John Galphin had driven off four hogs and killed or otherwise made away with them as he returned; the two men, Maubone Lubby, of Coweta, and Stimmauketah, of Tallahassee, asserting having set out on their return, with some salt, complained that the horses were poor and would not carry them home . . . ."

The role of salt as a trade item is illustrated by the following letter from Hawkins to one of the fur traders in the area:

"Cusseta, 26th of November, 1797: Auwihejee, son of Lauchejee, of Tallahassee, called on me for a letter to you; his father is called Crook Neck by our misnomers, and in that name I gave him a note to you. Lauchejee has 750 lbs of deer skins, and 36 lbs of beaver, which he takes down to you; his son, Auwihejee, and a black boy will accompany him. He leaves behind 200 deer skins and 30 or 40 small furs; these he will take down in the spring; for the value of these he wishes a credit till he can send them down.

"The goods he wants are 6 pcs Strouds, 1 pair white blankets and 1 pc Duffils, 3 pair arm bands, 3 pair wrist bands, 2 pcs petticoate linseys, 2 pcs white linen for shirts, 2 pcs black handkerchief, 2 or 3 pieces callico, 1 piece stripped cotton homespun, 1 piece negro cloth, 50 lbs powder and 100 lbs of lead,

12 fine combs, 12 long knives, 12 cutteaux knives, 12 pair scissars, ribband, binding, 1 lb white thread, 100 needles, flints, paint, 2 or 3 scarlet blankets, 3 pcs of romals, 3 pcs coarse check or stripe for shirts, 1 brass kettle, 7 bags salt, 1 keg of brandy, broaches, ear bobs, beads, 1 fowling piece, 1 hat, a good one, black feather; hatches, axes, looking glasses."

The use of salt as an item for the barter of Indian labor was quite familiar to the white settlers. In the course of his travels, Hawkins provided a vivid example of this practice:

"I took a view of Mr. Grierson's farm, he had planted the last season two acres of cotton in drills, 4 feet asunder; the land apparently not very good, high, dry and gravelly, the cotton grew well, many of the stalks 8 feet high . . . . He informs me he finds no difficulty in hiring the Indian women to pick out cotton, he hired them to pick by the basket of about a bushel, he gave half a pint of salt, or 3 strands of mock wampum beads a basket, or half a pint of taffra for 2 baskets; where the cotton was fully open, they could pick from two to three baskets the day."

The role occupied by salt in pacification of the Indians of the Creek Nation is highlighted by the meticulous itemization by Hawkins in his "Orders on Edward Price, U.S. Factor, for Sundries for the Creek Department as Contingencies." Salt was dispensed in quarts, bags and one-half bushel volumes. A short excerpt of the entries of January 4, 1798, illustrates this point:

"January 4, 1798: Iokee, 1 bag of salt.
John Barnard, 5 dollars.
Ohiethly Tustunnagau, 10 lbs of pork.
Ochese Tustunnagau, 9 bags of corn.
Emautlau Haujo, 1/2 bushel salt.

Tuskeegee Tustunnagau, 1 bushel of corn.
Suahoey, 30 lbs bacon.
Indian department, 1 bushel of corn.
Hothletocco, 2 bags of corn and 1 bag of salt."

Hawkins additionally dutifully recorded in his records the items distributed to individual Indians with bags of salt frequently noted. The dispersals chronologically given in his diary for the summer of 1798 substantiated this well:

"Creek Stipend for 1798

June 7 No. 1, Morgan of Wewokee, one bag of salt $1.00
23, 2, George Cornell, a chief of Tuckabatchee, for the use of the chiefs of the Creek nation: 100.00
Aug 17, 3, Nancy, the Indian woman under protection of the government: 318.1/2
One bag with flower and 20 lbs of beef.
21, 4, Haffocolotigee, her husband, and family one bag salt and one bag of 20 lbs flower 2.25
27, 5, Sohtigee, a Cusseta woman, one shift 150"

An additional description of the desire for salt by the Creek Indians was given by Hawkins in relation to a village near the Oconee River:

"Opoiuchee, of Sowgohatchee, applies for a trader in his town; he says there are thirty hunters and they will treat a white man well; that the women are in want of a man who will supply them with salt and thread for such articles of food as they can spare."

It would appear from these observations by Hawkins that no source of native salt was available to the Creek Indians. It further seems quite well documented that for at least some, more likely most, of this very large group, salt was not used in their pre-Columbian diet. It was only with the introduction of the concept of salting meat for purposes of preservation that salt became an important item of trade and pacification with the white man.

An additional recording of provision of salt to the Creek Nation appeared in the memoirs of de Milford (1956). In a discussion of the conflict between the Americans and the French in gaining favor and influence among the various Indian tribes, he quoted directly from an article which appeared in the *Gazette de* in 1802:

"The government of the United States seems to have already exceeded, up to a certain point, in its enterprise in civilizing the Indian tribes known as the Creeks, which are dispersed over the territory situated south of the Ohio. It has prevailed upon the natives of these districts to appoint six deputies from each tribe, who will meet in May every year to hold a national counsel . . . . The Indian deputies will eat and sleep in the building where the sittings are held and they will be furnished, at the expense of the American government, with beef, corn, beans, and salt."

The gift or barter of salt to the Indians by colonizing Europeans was not limited to those of English extraction. In the Spanish literature the inclusion of salt in the lists of gifts to the

Indians is detailed in a letter written by Alexander O'Reilly in 1770 (Bolton, 1914). At that time he was Commander of New Orleans and a large portion of the region ruled by the Spanish extending in all directions from the mouth of the Mississippi River. This correspondence, dated January 22, 1770, lists the effects to be given to four of the Indian nations (Grand Cados, Nachitos, Pequenos, Cados, and Yatasse) for their annual presents. For the Grand Cados and the Pequenos Cados, 25 pounds of salt were allotted each, while 20 pounds of the mineral were included in the list for the Yatasse Nation. None was allocated to the Nachitos. However, it is to be noted that several additional lists of annual gifts to various other Indian nations did not include salt. The absence may possibly be explained by these groups having access to salt of native manufacture (Bolton, 1914; Swanton, 1918-19).

The Choctaw Indians occupied a large extent of land located in the northern portions of the present-day states of Alabama and Mississippi roughly 300 miles above the entrance to Mobile Bay. There are scant accounts of the culture of this large group of Indians, but one French writer of the eighteenth century recorded in a handwritten narrative the most complete description in existence of the Choctaw domestic economy (Swanton, 1918-19)

"They have by way of furniture only an earthen pot in which to cook their food, some earthen pans for the same purpose, and some fanners or sieves and hampers to prepare their corn, which is their usual nourishment. They pound it in a wooden crusher (pile) or mortar, which they make out of the trunk of a tree, hollowed by means of burning embers. The pestle belonging to it is sometimes ten feet long and as small around as the arm. The upper end is an unshaped mass which serves to weigh it down and to give force to this pestle in falling back, in order to crush the corn more easily. After it is thus crushed they sift it in order to separate the finer part. They boil the coarser in a great skin which holds about three or four *sceau* of water, and mix it sometimes with pumpkins, or beans, or bean leaves. When this stew is almost cooked they throw into it the finest of the corn which they had reserved to thicken the water, and by way of seasoning they have a pot hung in the air in which are ashes of corn silk, beanpods, or finally oak ashes, on which having thrown water they take the lye which has fallen into a vessel provided underneath, and with it season their stew which is called *sagamite*. This serves as their principal food, and as well that of the French who are in the colony who have not the means of living otherwise.

"They sometimes make bread without lye, but rarely, because that consumes too much corn, and it is difficult to make, since they reduce it to flour only with the strength of their arms; after which it is kneaded or they boil it in water, or wrap it in leaves and cook it in the ashes, or finally having flattened the paste to the thickness of two crowns *(ecus)*, and the diameter of the two hands, they cook it on a piece of a pot on the embers. They also eat it with acorns. After having reduced the acorns to flour they put them in a cane sieve placed near the bank of a stream, and from time to time throw water upon them. By means of this lye they cause it to lose its bitterness after which they put the paste around a piece of wood which they cook in the fire. When they have meat they boil it in water, however dirty it is, without washing it, saying that that would make it lose its flavor. When it is cooked they sometimes put some of the acorn flour into the broth. They also cook unpounded corn with their meat, and when it is dry they pound it and reduce it to lint (*charpie*). They mix it in boiling with this corn. That has no taste and one must be a savage to eat it."

The above quite vividly describes the preparation of a form of condiment from the leaching of ashes derived from plant or wood sources. This practice was not unique and has been associated with unacculturated groups of both North and South America as well as natives of Oceania.

In the mid-nineteenth century, Henry R. Schoolcraft, in his capacity as the national Agent for Indian Affairs, was charged with preparing a report on the Indians of the continental United States. These reports appeared in a series of five lengthy volumes and described all aspects of the Indians, including a detailed account of their culture. In Volume II, published in 1852, Schoolcraft gave the following description of the Indians' preparation of foods:

"Roasting and boiling are simple operations for the Indian. There is no condiment to be used; no salt, no pepper. Soups are their great resource; particularly in seasons of want, or where the food would not admit of division by any other method. A squirrel, or a small bird, will answer to season or qualify a gallon of soup."

The reports of Schoolcraft identified all individual tribes, their geographic location, and estimates of population. The aforementioned description of the North American Indian appears to portray dietary customs among the vast majority of the Indian tribes inhabiting the middle continental United States.

In an account based upon 20 years of experience in contact with the Indians of the Great Plains and the mountains of the Far West continuing to the Pacific Ocean, Humfreville, a captain in the United States Cavalry, stated in his preface (1899):

"In this work I shall endeavor to give an accurate account of the daily life of the wild Indians, as I knew them in their native state. I have often been impressed with the fact that, both in their character and manner of life, they have been grossly misrepresented by modern writers, many of whom evidently depended upon vivid imaginations to furnish what personal experience and knowledge could not supply . . . . In the following chapters I shall describe the Indian as he was, when I first knew him, at which time he was absolutely a wild man . . . . It will be my aim to state the truth impartially, and nothing but the truth, to portray the Indian of fact, and not the Indian of fiction.

"Some apparent repetitions may be noticed in the text; but the reader must not forget that while the customs, characteristics, religious beliefs, and personal traits of the Indian nations and tribes were nearly identical in many respects, yet some of them differed in a variety of interesting ways. Hence in portraying the every day life of so many nations and tribes, I could not avoid at times a certain sameness of ideas and expressions, which, however, is more apparent than real."

In his description of the dietary habits of the Indians, Humfreville comments:

"When the Indian first came into intercourse with the white man, his most eager desire was to secure knives, hatchets, and kettles. He usually cooked his food by broiling it, or by semi-boiling it in a pot made of fresh hides or in hollowed wooden receptacles which answered the purpose of kettles. In these water was poured, and heated by hot stones which were constantly thrown in. When on the chase and hungry, he often ate his meat raw and bloody just as it was cut from the newly slain animal.

"As to taste, it did not figure at all in the Indians manner of preparing his food. His only thought was to appease his hunger, not to gratify his palate. Everything was cooked in miscellaneous fashion, a pot-pourri, or mess, which everybody partook while it lasted.

North America

"When food was scarce - for the Indian was the impersonation of improvidence - they would endure hunger uncomplainingly. When in desperate straights, they would eat skins, their moccasins, roots, buds, and the bark of trees were not despised. In times of want, as long as their ponies and dogs lasted, they did not fast long at a time. They didn't use salt with their food or as a condiment; they did not have it and were not accustomed to its use.

"In eating jerked meat, they rarely cooked it at all. It was left until thoroughly cured (in the sun), when the entire family could munch it all day."

Humfreville selected a number of Indian groups for detailed narrative. Among these were the Sioux nation. In his description of the dietary habits of the Sioux, he notes:

"The Sioux were carnivorous. They did not eat cereals, or vegetable food. They often ate their meat raw while the blood of the animal was still warm . . . . Commerce and trade were unknown to them . . . . When they had a pot or other vessel suitable to cook in, the meat was put into it and boiled. When they had no vessel, the meat was thrown on the coals and broiled, or held over the fire and roasted. The cooking, when in camp, was done by the women. If they had a pot it was always on the fire, and the contents were kept constantly boiling."

In his description of the Yurok Indians and other groups of the present-day northern California and Oregon regions, Humfreville provided a graphic description of the items of food collected by these tribes and their method of preparation. He noted:

"They preferred fishing to hunting, as it required less exertion . . . . Some of them caught fish by building closely constructed willow dams at certain places on the streams, so that the fish could not pass through; and when they swarmed at these dams, they were scooped out by means of baskets and drag-nets. Salmon especially were easily taken in this way by the northern tribes . . . . The coast Indians ate shell fish, seal, and stranded whales.

"Their principal food consisted of acorns and nuts. These were often eaten raw, or sometimes pounded into a pulp, then made into bread; this was baked in a hole in the ground, over which hot coals were heaped.

"Occasionally they ate their food raw; at other times it was half-boiled in close-woven baskets filled with water heated by hot stones. Meat was sometimes broiled or cooked in a hole in the ground, over which were placed live coals. The animal was roasted whole, just as it was killed, and entrails and all were eaten. They never washed their cooking utensils or their hands, although they uniformly ate with their fingers . . . . Fruits, roots, berries and vegetables formed part of their diet. The women did all of the fruit gathering, the men confined their labors to hunting and fishing. Some of the provident dried or smoked their fish and meats, and preserved roots, berries and acorns in baskets for seasons of want."

The Indians of the Columbia River area were described by Humfreville to depend principally upon hunting and fishing for food. He notes:

"Salmon and other fish were dried, then pulverized, and after being mixed with oil were laid away for winter use. Grasshoppers were secured by setting fire to the grass in dry weather and driving the insects into pits prepared for the purpose. At other times they formed a line and beat the ground with sticks, driving the grasshoppers into the pit. These insects, when caught in large numbers, were cooked in holes in the ground, over which fires were built; at other times they were dried and put away for future use, and when pulverized were made into a kind of paste or cake."

Cannibalism was not unknown among these tribes. Humfreville comments:

"Some tribes scalped their enemies, others did not. All were possessed of the innate Indian trait of torturing prisoners. They sometimes ate portions of the bodies of captives, not from a cannibalistic impulse, but to absorb the courage of the slain. Their wars, as a usual thing, were neither bloody nor prolonged. They invariably killed the male prisoners, and made slaves of captive women and children."

An approach to obtaining data which appears to be valid in reference to dietary intake of salt is the culture element distribution list utilized by Kroeber and colleagues in studies of 179 particular groups of Amerindians inhabiting the northwestern and southwestern areas of the United States (Kroeber, 1941). Several of the specific items in the list included use of salt and/or substances of high salinity. For each of the groups, it was determined whether mineral salt was used, the source of supply, whether seaweed was eaten, whether salt was manufactured by the roasting of selected grasses, and whether salt-taboo existed in the culture. This last item, if answered in the affirmative, would indicate that the group considered salt or substances of high salinity to be desirable and that exclusion of the use of salt during a ritual would provide further substantiation of its routine use within that society.

In an initial presentation of selected data obtained from the culture element distribution list study, Kroeber described the distribution of the use of salt and of substances of high salinity for the 279 groups. Of note was the observation that salt was used, almost without exception, in the southern half of the study area and not used, almost without exception, in the northern portion of the study area (Figure II-1). The identified line of geographic demarcation for this dietary characteristic commenced on the Pacific shore at the mouth of the Columbia River, then proceeded south to the California/Oregon border, subsequently cutting southeasterly to reach its most southern point between Walker and Carson Lakes of mid-Nevada. The dividing line then swung north to southeastern Oregon and lastly turned eastward across the Snake River. Kroeber identified these nine tribes to be non-salt users: Chinook, Tenino, Klamath, Modoc, Eastern Achoawi, Paiute, Lemhi, Soshone, and Chilcotin. These represent specific tribes identified to be living geographically at the most southern reaches of the borderline separating non-salt users from salt users. Of note is the fact that these Indians not only did not use mineral salt, they did not use other sources of high salinity, including seaweed or minerals manufactured by roasting of particular grasses (*Distichlis spicata* - a salt grass inhabiting salt marshes and alkaline soil along the coast and in certain interior valleys and deserts of the southern extent of the study). Within the central portion of the area identified with non-salt users are located the following additional ten tribes: Thompson, Jutenai, Wenatchi, Sanpoil, Kalispel, Kitittas, Klikitat, Coeur d-Alene, Flathead, and Wada-dökadö. As noted, with rare exception, other groups living within the no-salt region were identified also to be non-salt users. Thus, the report of Kroeber substantiates that a minimum of 19 specific tribes or groups were identified by the culture element distribution technique to constitute no-salt cultures.

In a contemporary observation, an additional group of Indians living in the western sub-arctic areas of North America have been identified to have existed in a no-salt culture (Helm, 1972). She noted that the Dogrib Indians and neighboring tribes north of Great Slave Lake never had access to sodium chloride (1979). She commented that prior to the introduction of flour, lard, and a few other comestibles about 100 years ago, the Dogribs were almost exclusively fish and mammal-flesh eaters. The exception was the availability of several species of berries only during the month of August. She stated:

"It is my impression, from when I began work with the neighboring Slave tribe in 1951, that even up to 1950 most families never bought salt at the trading post. By a few years later, however, one Dogrib commented to me that 'We are just like white men now,' as he reached for the salt shaker."

She further commented:

"To my knowledge there is only one source of 'natural' salt anywhere in the broad basin of the Athabaskan tribes of the north. This is on the Salt River south of the Great Slave Lake. This river is completely outside of Dogrib territory; there is no evidence in any of the literature that salt was ever taken from that deposit by the Chipewyan tribes of that region either for their own purposes or for trade to other tribes. For none of the tribes, Dogrib included, was salt (even to the present day) used for the preservation of meat or fish."

Turning to the northern continent, the Eskimos of the North American continent were basically a carnivorous race in their unacculturated state. A list of the components of their diet includes the caribou, arctic hare, fox, muskox, polar bear, seal, whale, walrus, ptarmigan, fish, and numerous sea birds including geese, duck, hawk, gulls, and a variety of others. One of the few exceptions to the general description of the Eskimo eating all portions of the animals, including the intestines, is the liver of the polar bear which contains a toxic concentration of vitamin A. Of note, even the dogs leave this particular portion of the bear untouched.

Primitive Peoples Without Salt

One of the earlier observations of dietary characteristics of Eskimos living in the region of Frobisher Bay is provided by Hall (1865). He described vividly the behavior of the Eskimos following the killing of a Greenland whale (Mysticetus):

"The skin of the *Mysticetus* (Greenland whale) is a great treat to the Esquimaux, who eat it raw; and even before the whale was brought to the ship, some of the skin, about twenty square feet, had, by permission, been consumed by hungry natives. The 'black skin' is three fourths of an inch thick, and looks like India-rubber. It is good eating in its raw state even for a white man, as I know from experience; but when boiled and soused in vinegar it is most excellent.

"I afterward saw the natives cutting up the *krang* (meat) of the whale into such huge slices as their wives could carry; and as they worked, so did they keep eating.

"As I stood upon the rocky shore observing the busy natives at work carving the monster before me, my eye caught a group around one of the vertebrae, from which they were slicing and eating thin pieces of ligament that looked white and delicious as the breast of a Thanksgiving turkey! At once I made up my mind to join in partaking of the inviting (?) viands actually smoking in my sight. Taking from the hands of Ugarng his seal-knife, I peeled off a delicate slice of this spinal ligament, closed my eyes, and cried out 'Turkey!' But it would not go down so easy. Not because the stomach has posted up its sentinel to say 'no whale can come down here' but because it was tougher than any bull beef of Christendom! For half an hour I tried to masticate it, and then found it was even tougher than when I began. At length I discovered I had been making a mistake in the way to eat it. The Esquimaux custom is to get as vast a piece into their distended mouths as they can cram, and then, boa constrictor-like, first lubricate it over, and so swallow it quite whole!

"One old woman kindly came to me and offered a generous slice of the 'whalegum' she was feasting on. Reaching out my hand, with one stroke of her '*ood-loo*' (a woman's knife - an instrument like a mincing knife) she severed the white, fibrous strip quick as thought. It cut as old cheese. Its taste was like unripe chestnuts, and its appearance like cocoa-nut meat. But I can not say this experiment left me a very great admirer of whale's gum, though, if the struggle was for life, and its preservation depended on the act, I would undoubtedly eat whale's gum until I got something better to my liking."

Hall further described his participation in a feast of freshly killed raw seal. This occurred in an Eskimo tent made of skins:

"Bowing down almost to a horizontal position, in went head, shoulders, body, and all. The next second I found myself butt up against a dozen Esquimaux, all lusty fellows, and crowded together in a heap, each armed with a knife! But there was no cause for alarm. The knives were not for any warlike or evil purpose. They were being used simply for cutting off strips of seal, to be shoved into the widely-extended mouths of the hungry people before me. Quite at the back of the tent I perceived my Esquimaux friend Koojesse seated between two pretty females, all three engaged in doing full justice to a dish of smoking-hot seal-blood! Seeing me, Koojesse at first seemed abashed; but, on my expressing a readiness to partake of any food they had to spare, one of the women immediately drew forth from the stew-pan about four inches of seal vertebrae, surrounded by good meat. I managed to eat the latter, and then determined to try the seal-blood. To my surprise, I found it excellent.

"The first thing done was to consecrate the seal, the ceremony being to sprinkle water over it, when the stalwart host and his assistant proceeded to separate the 'blanket' - that is, the blubber, with skin - from the solid meat and skeleton of the seal. The body was then opened and the blood scooped out. This blood is considered very precious, and forms an important item of the food largely consumed by Esquimaux. Next came the liver, which was cut into pieces and distributed all around, myself getting and eating a share. Of course it was eaten raw - for this was a raw-meat feast - its eating being accompanied by taking into the mouth at the same time a small portion of delicate white blubber, which answered the same as butter with bread. Then followed distributing the ribs of the seal for social picking. I joined in all this, doing as they did, and becoming quite an Innuit save in the quantity eaten. This I might challenge any white man to do. No human stomach but an Innuit's could possibly hold what I saw these men and women devour."

In a further portion of his account, Hall described living alone with a group of Innuit Eskimos for 42 days in an igloo and existing primarily upon their native food. During this time he described his participation in the Eskimo life pattern of feast or famine with the entire village, including Hall, without food for more than four days when a seal was finally killed.

In 1922, Stefansson more precisely discussed the Eskimo and salt. In presenting the experiences of his colleague, Dr. Anderson, with the Mackenzie Eskimo in the Yukon Valley, Stefansson stated:

"During the four months that intervened between this and our next meeting he secured numerous specimens of sheep, caribou, and other far northern mammals, and incidentally had his first experience of 'living on the country.' . . . It was, incidentally, Dr. Anderson's first experience of living without salt, an ordeal which he had much dreaded, for he shared the common belief that salt is a necessary article of diet. But it turned out, as I knew from experience it would, that he did not mind it seriously.

"Most people are in the habit of looking upon the articles of our accustomed diet, and especially upon salt, as necessities. We have not found them so. The longer you go without grain foods and vegetables the less you long for them. Salt I have found to behave like a narcotic poison - in other words, it is hard to break off its use, as it is hard to stop the use of tobacco; but after you have been a month or so without salt you cease to long for it, and after six months I have found the taste of meat boiled in salt water distinctly disagreeable. In the case of such a necessary element of food as fat, on the other hand, I have found that the longer you are without it the more you long for it, until the craving becomes much more intense than is the hunger of a man who fasts. (The symptoms of starvation are of a disease rather than of being hungry.) Among the uncivilized Eskimo the dislike of salt is so strong that a saltiness imperceptible to me would prevent them from eating at all. This circumstance was often useful to me later in our travels about Coronation Gulf, for whenever our Eskimo visitors threatened to eat us out of house and home we could put in a little pinch of salt, and thus husband our resources without seeming inhospitable. A man who tasted anything salty at our table would quickly bethink him that he had plenty of more palatable fare in his own house."

Actual measurements of urinary electrolytes in samples obtained from Eskimos are limited to determinations of urinary chloride. The subjects for the study constituted Eskimos living on the islands of South Hampton, Baffin, Devon, and Ellesmere north of the Hudson Bay (Rabinowitch, 1936; 1937). Until introduced by Canadians, this investigator noticed that the Eskimos of the Canadian Eastern Arctic had no salt in their diets beyond the quantities of that mineral naturally present in their basically carnivorous diet. In his reports of clinical and metabolic observations of these Eskimos, Rabinowitch included measurements of plasma and urinary concentrations of chloride in 22 subjects representing five groups living on the four islands. The results were expressed as percent concentration of sodium chloride, even though the former ion was not measured. Plasma chloride concentrations were interpreted to be high with mean values of 603 mg/dl which, when converted to mEq, give a mean value of 103.9 mEq/l. In respect to urinary values, the mean concentration of chloride expressed as sodium chloride was 0.175 mg/dl with the lowest value of .02 mg/dl. These represent 31 and 3.4 mEq/l respectively on these urine samples collected from the 22 subjects.

Interpretation of these data in respect to urinary concentration of sodium requires some caution. In our investigation of the Yanomamö Indians in whom urinary concentrations of sodium averaged approximately 1 mEq/l, simultaneous determinations of urinary chloride often gave marked discrepancies in concentrations (Oliver, 1975; Oliver, unpublished data). For although the excretion of these two ions may parallel in some individuals in whom the urinary concentration of sodium is 1 mEq/l, simultaneous concentrations of urinary chloride exceeded 75 mEq/l in some samples and rarely were less than 6 mEq/l. Obviously, the dietary patterns of Eskimos and of South American Indians are markedly dissimilar, but these data raise the possibility that the concentrations of urinary sodium could be much lower than those estimated by determination of urinary chloride only. Inasmuch as the specific gravity of the urine samples averaged 1.015 with densities ranging between 1.010 and 1.024, Rabinowitch concluded that the findings regarding urinary chloride were not spurious as a consequence of dilute samples. In discussion of his findings, he suggested that the low urinary output of chloride, expressed as sodium chloride, matched the dietary habits of the Eskimos who have an absence of sodium chloride in their diet beyond that naturally present in their native foods.

It is thus possible to state through reports of those initially contacting a significant number of tribes of North American Indians and groups of Eskimos that a large proportion of the indigenous population could be accurately described to have been no-salt cultures at the time of the intitial post-Columbian contact with Europeans. The general impression is gained that the introduction of salt and its various uses as a condiment and as a preservative quickly followed colonization in North America. Simultaneously, however, other groups living on the same continent used salt as a standard commodity. Exploration of possible reasons to account for this dichotomy consitutes a subsequent chapter.

The distribution of these 'no-salt' groups is depicted in Figure II-2. Cultures living in diverse environmental circumstances without salt were clearly in the majority throughout the North American continent.

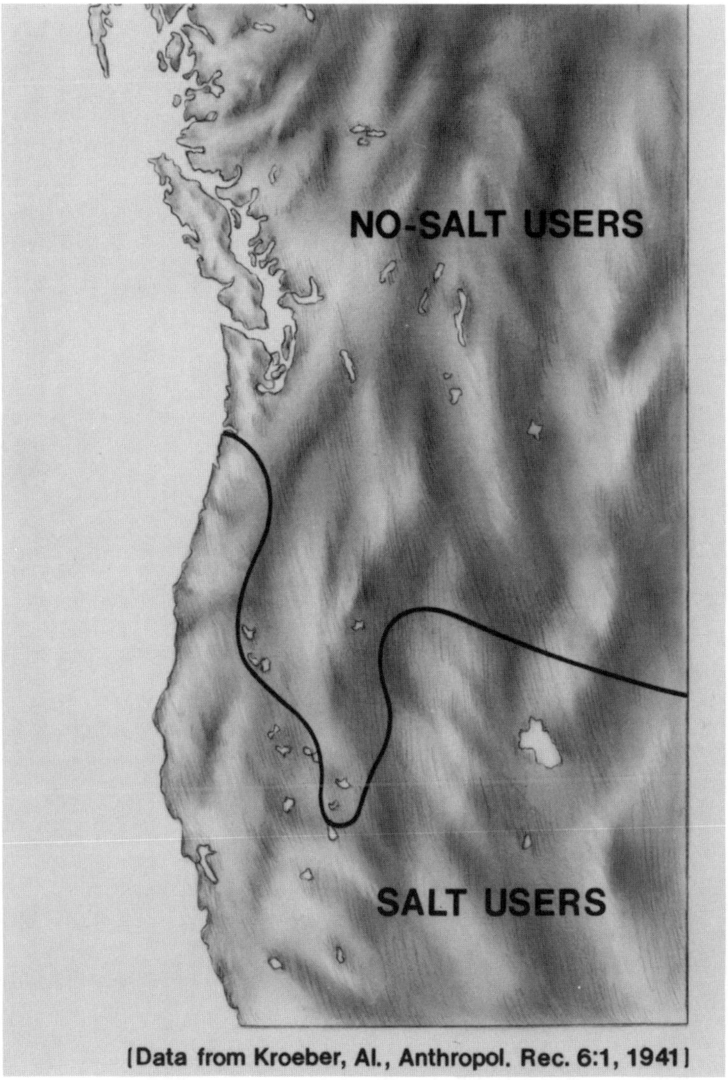

Figure: II-1: Location of 'No-Salt Users' and 'Salt-Users' among Amerindians of western North America.

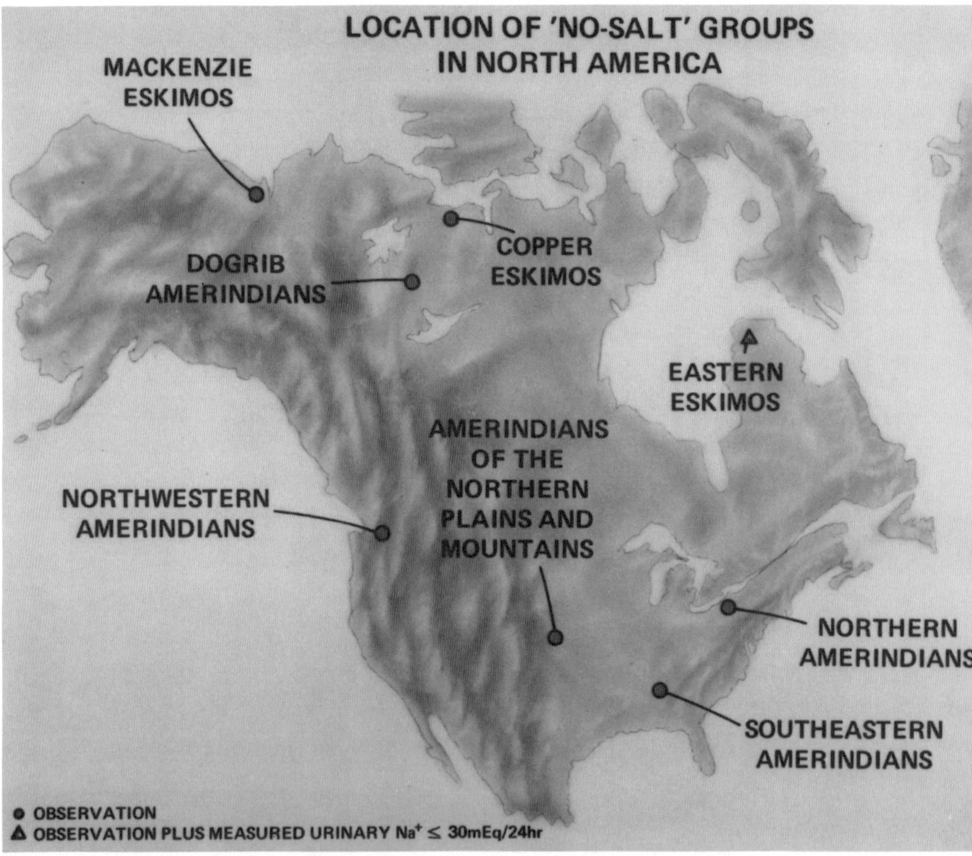

Figure: II-2: Location of 'No-Salt' Groups in North America.

North America

III. South America

Publications regarding dietary customs related to salt among the Amerindians of South America vary from reported observations to studies in which timed urine collections have been analyzed for sodium and other constituents These latter investigations have been also combined with measurements of the major sodium-related hormones.

An early account of a tribe subsisting without salt was recorded by Schomburgk (1840-1844) in his description of the Warrau Indians living on the banks of the Barima River in present day Guyana:

"Game and fish constitute their chief nourishment, though they do not disdain rats, monkeys, alligators, frogs, worms, caterpillars, larvae and beetles. They are surprisingly adept in catching fish, which they capture partly with hooks, partly with bow and arrow, or kill with light spears. If the capture proves greater than the requirement, some of them will sun-dry the surplus and bring it to town for sale, but such industrious ones are only rarely met with. Meat, under these skies, turns bad within two or three hours, and if they want to keep it a while for further use so that, released from the chase, they can enjoy undistrubed rest, they build a small staging about four-foot high with cross pieces resting on the top of the four corner-posts stuck into the ground: they spread the flesh on this, the women keeping up a moderate fire beneath it for from 20 to 24 hours. By this means the meat keeps good for some 5 to 6 days, but dry and without nourishment - this is especially the case with four-footed animals." . . .Game is cooked in the blood of the animal, and strongly seasoned with Capsicum*."

A more vivid personal experience occurred in 1907 when

---

*A variety of pepper.

a young novice Peruvian *cauchero* (rubber tree tapper) was abducted by hunters of the Amahuacas Amerindians. The village of this tribe was located near the head-waters of the Purus River, a southwestern tributary of the Amazon River on the border between Brazil and Peru. The captured youth was adopted into the tribe and lived continuously with these unacculturated natives for over two and one-half years. In his autobiography, Cordova-Rios (1971) wrote:

"After perhaps six months with the *Huni Kui* (meaning the Chosen People) I had become accustomed to living in the nude, to eating their unsalted diet of jungle game, the few products of their primitive agriculture and wild fruit. And I understood a few words of their strange vocabulary."

Two years later, Cordova-Rios successfully reached an isolated jungle trading post with blocks of *caucho* (rubber) produced by his Amerindian comrades to barter for guns, ammunition, machetes, knives, and beads. He described the lunch given him by the Brazilian traders:

"We ate Brazilian bean stew, *feijoada completa,* a complete meal with farina to mix with the rice, beans and meat. All this was followed by sweet black coffee. The food tasted good, and it reminded me of my past."

Further in the narrative of this venture, he detailed his indigestion during the return trip with his Indian companions to the village:

"As we moved through the forest I became increasingly aware of distress in my stomach. When we stopped at midmight I was in trouble with diarrhea. For over two years I had eaten nothing seasoned with salt and felt that this and the unaccustomed food must have caused my upset. My companions were immediately suspicious of poison, but I assured them there was no reason to be.

"In the morning they prepared an herbal concoction for me to drink, and it helped my distress. We went on, but I was weak. After my system cleared completely of salt and my food was again limited to smoked meat and fruit from the forest, my condition improved."

Cordova-Rios later escaped from his captors. Subsequently, his knowledge of forest plants led him to a renowned career as a medicine man and as a consultant for commercial exploration of medicinal plants.

A more formal and detailed description of the Siriono Indians of eastern Bolivia was made by Holmberg (1950). The Siriono at the time of his observations were semi-nomadic groups who subsisted primarily by hunting, fishing, and gathering supplemented by a minimal degree of primitive agriculture. These Indians were considered to have been at the Paleolithic level of culture. The Siriono had lost the art of making fire and by necessity carried fire from one campsite to the next. Regarding salt, Holmberg noted. that:

"The Siriono, moreover, have no salt with which to preserve meat, nor have they developed any techniques of drying and smoking meat to render it edible for more than two or three days. . . . No condiments of any kind are used in cooking, even salt (no deposits of this product are found in the area) is unknown to the Siriono living under aboriginal conditions. Evidently, the foods they eat contain enough salt to produce the hydrochloric acid necessary for digestion."

Holmberg further described the response of these Indians to their first exposure to salt:

"I introduced salt to some Indians for the first time, and they expressed a distaste for eating it. By using small quantities in cooking, however, they soon developed a craving for it. In some instances this craving (once the Indians have become accustomed to using salt) has become so great as to become an important factor in establishing and maintaining friendly relations with the whites. The late Frederick Park Richards, an American cattle rancher living near El Carmen, who was one of the first white men to establish permanent relations with the Siriono in the Rio Blanco area, told me that when he first came to the region in 1912 he was able to maintain peaceful relations with the Indians for years before they permanently settled down with him on his farms in 1925 by conditioning them to eating salt. I myself, however, have traveled with primitive groups when all of us went without salt for as long as 43 days without suffering any apparent ill effects from such a diet."

In the course of a nutrition survey, Lowenstein (1961) measured the blood pressure of members of two tribes of Brazilian Indians living in the Amazon Basin of northern Brazil. One tribe, the Carajas, were considered by the investigator to be quite primitive. The other, the Mundurucus, had moved into a mission village some four decades previously. In discussing the higher blood pressure values associated with increasing age of representatives of the latter tribe, Lowenstein noted:

"There have been other changes in their life habits - e.g., the regular use of table salt (sodium chloride) instead of plant ashes (potassium chloride) and the use of tobacco."

The Waorani Amerindians are a group of slightly over 600 individuals living in the largely unexplored headwaters of the upper Amazon Basin south of the Rio Napo in eastern Ecuador (Larrick, 1979). The persistent hostility of the group toward outsiders resulted in a delay of contact until the late

1950's for a portion of the group while the remainder have been contacted only since 1968. The Waorani represent an inter-riverine group of the tropical rain forest culture. Linguistically, they are an isolate; no affiliation with any other South American language has been identified. Initially, they were unskilled in canoe building, had no knowledge of swimming, and totally avoided large rivers when on spearing raids against outsiders.

The major portion of the native Waorani diet was obtained from subsistence agriculture which provided most of their carbohydrates, while dietary protein was obtained primarily from hunted game or fish. The largest single component of their diet consisted of manioc (*Manihot utilissima*) which was consumed in large quantities as a premasticated drink. Other cultivated crops included corn, peanuts, plantains, and sweet potatoes. Supplementation to the diet was provided by wild fruits, nuts, and tubers gathered during travels through the tropical rain forest. The traditional diet of the Waorani contained no salt. Doctor Larrick (1982) noted:

"There was no consumption or trade of exogenous salt. Some plants and the meat may have supplied sodium chloride."

Although indigenous peanuts consitututed one of their standard crops, he observed that when offered salted peanuts these were immediately spat out by the Waorani as unpalatable food! However, Doctor Larrick further commented (1982):

"The people are currently consuming outside food which is often heavily salted."

In the course of multidisciplinary biomedical studies, it was concluded that the Waorani Indians were healthy individuals. Physical examinations of 60 percent of the total population substantiated that the people in general were well-nourished, without anemia, and represented a population in which blood pressure did not increase with age. The Waorani are physically very active people. The anthropometric data indicated an absence of obese individuals. The investigators provided several reasons for the perceived good health of the Waorani. Diet was considered to be adequate with sufficient vitamins, carbohydrates, and protein while low in salt and animal fat. The isolation until the past decade served to protect these Amerindians from the introduction of diseases noted for causing high morbidity and mortality among primitive groups (Neel, 1970).

The absence of salt or substances of high salinity in the diet has not resulted in a lack of population expansion. Based on birth rates obtained since the Waorani were first contacted in 1968, annual growth rate of the population has been estimated to be 2.2 percent. Data indicated a completed fertility of 5.7 births per woman.

The indigenous culture of the Waorani thus appears to have resulted in good general health and in annual population expansion. In fact, the major cause of demise of both male and female Indians was homocide by others of the tribal group.

The Guayaki Amerindians of the inland tropical rain forest of eastern Paraquay have inhabited the same territory for an undetermined number of centuries (Clastres, 1972). First identification of the Guayaki as a distinct group was described in the eighteenth century in the writings of the Jesuit priest, Father Pedro Lozano (1874). The territory of these Amerindians was inclusively within the right bank of the Parana River to the east, the Sierra de Mbaracaju to the north, and the Andean Belt of Caaguazu and the Sierra de San Joaquin to the west. This region, which was characterized by many large and small streams, was the watershed between the tributaries of the right bank of the Parana River and the tributaries of the left bank of the Paraquay River. The Guayaki Amerindians who have been studied extensively by Clastres are described as nomadic hunters living successfully in a roving existence within the tropical rain forest. Their isolation to the middle of the twentieth century is emphasized by the lack of sustained contact and comprehensive observation until late in the 1950's.

The indigenous technology of the Guayaki was restricted to those skills and tools appropriate to sustain a nomadic hunting society. For the men, equipment consisted of bows and various types of arrow, the latter dependent upon the object of the hunt, stone hatchets, hardwood lances, and digging sticks. For the women, the ubiquitous basket was carried across the back and secured to a wide frontal headband and contained the paucity of household items essential for sustenance. These included sleeping mats, feathers for new arrows for their husbands, earthenware pots for cooking or for storage of food, and knives derived from monkey fibulae and slivers of bamboo. Although the Guayaki made fire with friction utilizing two pieces of wood, it was far less effort for the women to carry a piece of live coal from one campsite to the next.

Bands of the Guayaki tended to number between 15 and 20. These numbers provided enough males for protection against other groups and simultaneously increased the likelihood that sufficient food would be found for needs of the entire band. The bands moved usually in forest areas of at least 300 square miles in the course of their nomadic search for food.

For the Guayaki, the tropical forest provided a smorgasbord. It has been noted by Clastres that:

"The life of the Guayaki depends directly upon a familiarity with their natural habitat, and it should be added here that these Indians eat all animals of the forest, almost without exception. Only a small number of birds which serve an important mythological function are not used for food.

"The animals killed most often by the Guayaki, be they big or small, are wild pigs, deer, coatis, armadillos, iguanas, capivaras, agoutis, jaguars, ant-eaters , and monkeys. Various sorts of rats, serpents, lizards and most types of birds which are found in such large numbers thoughout the South American forest are also killed, such as birds of prey, partridges, pheasants, vultures, and even small birds, which when plucked in the wink of an eye and quicky roasted are crunched in one mouthful. It is nearly useless to give a complete list of the animals the Guayaki kill because they eat everything."

Gathering complements hunting, but observers have considered the Paraguayan forest to be poor in consumable vegetation. Marrow of the palm tree and fibers of its trunk were made into a coarse flour. A boiled mixture of this flour with various larvae was made into soup and was a much favored delicacy. Larvae of multiple species were avidly sought, but the larvae (*guchu*) of the Coleoptera (*Mynda*), which were often up to four inches in length and rich in fat, were eaten with relish either raw or cooked. Even nursing infants were fed these larvae after the hard head had been removed with maternal fingernails. In fact, this was perhaps the only form of cultivating by these Indians in that palm trees were deliberately cut into sections of 10 to 12 feet facilitating the deposition of eggs by the insects. Each man was the owner of his larva bed. The domain of this private property was always respected, but the gathered harvest was divided and eaten collectively. For the nomadic Guayaki, preparation of the palm trees for deposition of eggs established a fixed source of food for gathering at a later time. Although this return was often many months later, the anticipated availability of these larvae at different sites exerted a profound influence upon the wandering habits of these Amerindians in providing an orderly pattern to their nomadic travels.

The food practices of the Guayaki have been described by Claustres:

"There is no apparent order in the hour of the Indian meal. One eats when one is hungry. It seems, however, that the evening meal is the most consistent of the day. This is understandable, since the day is generally spent hunting food that will be eaten in the evening.

"Cooking is, of course, a task that falls to the women. It is rudimentary, and the meat is either boiled in earthenware pots or roasted. Monkey meat, for example, is always boiled (*baku*); venison or wild pig is always roasted (*kai*). The game is sometimes poorly cooked, and often the repugnant odor of half-spoiled armadillo meat comes from the women's baskets. When some large game is killed (deer, jaguar, horse, or cow), it is cut into quarters to be roasted on a large wooden grill (*byta*), under which a fire burns. Moreover, the cutting up and dismembering of the game is subject to numerous prohibitions, depending upon the animals. For example, a man cannot without great danger cut up an armadillo--his wife must do it. Likewise, each person eats only certain meats or certain parts of the animals. Thus a woman pregnant with her first child should not eat the meat of the howling monkey; or a man in his prime should not suck from the head of an animal, which is reserved for old people. As for the huge larvae of certain large insects, they are not only eaten raw but also alive. The meat is torn with the bare hands, and the juice which flows down the fingers is sucked with pleasure. The delicious marrow of the pindo palm is generally eaten as soon as it is obtained, but the women also know how to make a kind of thick soup out of it (*bruee*), to be eaten with larvae. The Guayaki know nothing about salt, fermented drinks, or tobacco. Their food is marked by one great contrast: the sweet, or sugared (*ee*), and the bitter (*iro*). The Guayaki hate the bitter and are very fond of sweets, of which honey is an example."

It would appear from the sketchy historical data available that the Guayaki have remained within their present-day territory since the conquest of Paraguay by the Spaniards. However, the Guayaki's fear of their neighbors, the Mbya-Guarani and of the colonizing Paraguayans led to their intentional isolation until only the last several decades. The survival of this tribe and its descendants to present day without knowledge or use of salt appears quite well documented.

The Kayapo Amerindians of the southeastern Brazilian rain forests have been the subjects of biomedical studies directed to elucidating prehistoric epidemic disease patterns (Black, 1980). In the course of investigating noninfectious diseases, mean diastolic blood pressures were found to be significantly lower in 300 male and female Kayapo Amerindians than those of Northern American subjects of comparable age groups.

In response to specific inquiry, Dr. Black noted (1981):

"These are data (blood pressure measurements) from the Xikrin, Mekranoti and two Parakana villages. I never saw salt imported to these villages, nor saw it used by the Indians. Their food certainly tastes very saltless. I was told they could make salt from wood ash but this did not seem to be a regular procedure. The Kayapo tribes cook much of their food by roasting in the coals -- they have no ceramics -- and ingest considerable ash that way. I would not doubt that salt has been imported but it is not a regular trade item."

The observations appear to convincingly describe a no-salt culture. These Amerindians differed culturally from the

Waorani and were similar to the Guayaki in representing pre-agricultural societies (Black, 1980).

As part of an international cooperative investigation of electrolytes and blood pressure (INTERSALT), members of 10 native tribes in the *Parque Indigena do Zingus* of central Brazil were studied (Carvalho, 1989). Adults were chosen by random sampling of subjects from the 10 tribes. The diet of all groups consisted principally of manioc (*cassava*) and fish. Lesser components of the diet included corn, sweet potatoes, cara, peanuts, bananas, and wild fruit. Meat intake was sporadic. The authors stated that salt and other foods were sold in neighborhood stores but not used regularly. Dietary sodium and potassium were assessed by measurement of 24-hour urinary excretion. The results for sodium excretion were 13.6±25.2 (SD) mEq per 24 hours for 99 men and 11.0± 17.0 (SD) mEq per 24 hours for 99 women. For potassium, the values were 95.6± 40.8 (SD) per 24 hours and 78.5± 46.0 (SD) per 24 hours for the men and women, respectively. The investigators concluded that these subjects had a median intake of one third gram of salt daily. From descriptions of the customary diet and the measured urinary electrolyte excretions, it appears highly likely that an original native diet with minimum salt content was contaminated with some small frequent quantities of salt and salt-containing foods.

The Yanomamö Amerindians inhabiting the tropical equatorial rain forest of northern Brazil and southern Venequela have been the subjects for our studies of a no-salt culture (Oliver, 1975; Oliver, 1981). Since our investigations included several approaches and biomedical measurements not included in other studies of no-salt and low-salt cultures, our findings will be presented in some depth to provide a perspective for considering data from studies of other groups.

Some 12,000 to 15,000 Yanomamö Amerindians are distributed among 150 or more villages over an area exceeding 100,000 square miles (Figure III-1). Although briefly contacted by various explorers, sustained contact with any of the villages of this tribe dates back only to the early 1950's when missionary posts began to be established. The accumulated genetic and linguistic data indicate that the Yanomamö Amerindians have had a high degree of isolation for at least the past several thousand years (Neel, 1972). This is additionally emphasized by the distinct uniqueness of their intestinal flora (Eveland, 1971) and the absence of serum antibodies to ubiquitous viruses (measles) (Neel, 1970).The topography of the land inhabited by the Yanomamö ranges from villages located at near sea level altitude, with constant oppressively hot days broken by frequent tropical rain showers, to villages located at altitudes of 500 feet, nestled in mountainous areas where peaks exceed altitudes of 7,500 feet. In these latter villages, daytime temperatures approach the mid-nineties, but evenings are characteristically cool. Rainfalls are frequent, and the vegetation is lush and plentiful. In our investigations, subjects were selected from different villages at varying altitudes and a cross-section of dispersed geographic sites in Brazil and Venezuela, as remote as possible but still accessible by small boat and/or plane. The findings were similar in all the natives to whom government workers, missionaries, or traders had not introduced salt.

The subsistence of the Yanomamö can be characterized as consisting of slash-and-burn agriculture (Figure III-2), supplemented by the irregular addition of game, fish, insects, and wild vegetable foods (Oliver, 1975). The principal staple is the cooking banana, *musa paradisica* (Figures III-3 and III-4), which is cultivated with manioc and taro (Figure III-5). Hames (1980) estimated that cultivated foods provided 75 to 80 percent of the caloric intake. Similar dietary characteristics have been described also by Good (1987). The Yanomamö had no domesticated animals, except for dogs. These were highly valued for their protective deterrence against unexpected raids by warriors from other Yanomamö villages (Figure III-6). For protein, they relied on animals obtained by hunting and fishing. Chagnon and Hames (1979) interpreted their observations of game capture to be consistent with an intake of animal protein well exceeding the highest levels recommended by the National Research Council (1974). The authors cautioned that success of hunting by the Yanomamö was highly variable and several days could pass without meaningful additions of meat to the diet.

In their pre-contacted culture, the Yanomamö had no access to sodium chloride nor substances of high salinity. It was not a trade item, and their initial exposure to salt followed its introduction by government workers, missionaries, and, later, traders commencing with contacts first in the early 1950's. By prior inquiry, we excluded for these studies all villages in which salt had been introduced.

The language of the Yanomamö had no native word for salt. The word which they acquired for the mineral was *sayu*, which was derived from the Spanish or Portugese word *sal* corrupted into *sayu* because the Yanomamö could not terminate words with the speech sounds / -r / = / -l / (Chagnon, 1980). For seasoning, the Yanomamö used a "bush salt." A description of the preparation and use of this material has been provided by Chagnon who lived and worked for over two decades in villages of previously uncontacted Yanomamö (Chagnon, 1980). He noted:

"Their equivalent (to sodium chloride) as a condiment is a liquid made by (1) burning the bark of a species of tree (a palm, I believe), and then (2) leaching the ashes with water to yield a liquid, quite dirty and ash-filled, into which they dunk the food that they like to season this way. . . . . . I have seen them make it and use it on camping trips, and tasted it myself. It does resemble salt in a vague way insofar as taste goes."

No analyses of samples of this bark ash preparaton have been made; but from analyses of "bush salt" from other localities, it is highly unlikely to contain much, if any, sodium salts (McKee, 1955). Chagnon further commented:

"When given salt (sodium chloride) for the first time, the Yanomamö are often repulsed by its severe taste. They rapidly become avid, and eagerly seek it out once they have become accustomed to it."

For the Yanomamö prior to contact with outsiders, the major source of sodium was the various game that constituted part of their diet. A wide variety of animals were hunted, including anteaters, armadillos, capybara, deer, monkeys, peccaries, rodents, tapir, birds, snakes, freshwater crayfish, plus various insects. Opportunistic additions were seldom rejected (Figures III-7 and III-8). Fish constituted another source of sodium in their diet.

During a field expedition in 1987, food and other samples were collected and subsequently analyzed for their content of minerals and nutrients. As would be anticipated, the analyses confirmed a paucity of sodium in the non-animal sources of food (Table III-1). However, field observations which were subsequently confirmed by laboratory analyses identified two additional sources of dietary sodium. It is customary for the Yanomamö to roast raw vegetables, i.e., peeled plantains, and many other forms of food, directly in the hot cooking ashes which adhere to the food and are consumed without hesitation or apparent distaste (Figure III-9). These same cooking ashes are mixed with the native tobacco which is chewed daily by men, women, and older children (Figure III-10). The content of the cooking ashes varied considerably in the quantity of sodium present with a range of 1.85 mg to 271.32 mg of sodium per 100 grams of the original sample (Table III-2). The wide diversity of sodium content of the native wood probably reflects differing quantities of that ion in the soil, as well as characteristics of the various species of trees. Inasmuch as the Yanomamö are not selective in their collection of firewood, it is not surprising that significant variation was found. Nevertheless, these analyses confirmed a possible contribution of wood ashes to dietary sodium intake from the residuum accidentally adherent to food, as well as the quantity intentionally mixed with the chewing tobacco.

The practice of endocannibalism by the Yanomamö serve as an unusual, but a likely insignificant, source of sodium salts (Chagnon, 1980). Bodies of the dead are burned upon a pyre of wood, and the ashes sifted to permit collection of all pieces of bone and teeth. Following pulverization, the resultant powdered bones are consumed entirely (if an infant) or placed into small, hollow gourds (if an adult). In either case, at the time of consumption, a thick soup made of ripened plantains serves as a vehicle for the ashes and the mixture drunk. Ashes of infants and those of adults not dying in warfare are consumed by both sexes. Remains of men slain in warfare are never consumed immediately by other men. These ashes are used in pre-raid rituals and only totally consumed after the death has been avenged even if years later.

In the environment of the Yanomamö Amerindians, observations and analyses substantiated sodium to be a scarce dietary mineral. But, obviously, there is a minimum physiological requirement for sodium which must be met in some manner by these people. As noted earlier, the most likely major source of sodium in view of the characteristics of their diet was the meat of animal and fish origin. It is of interest to attempt to quantify the dietary sodium associated with consumption of meat. Chagnon and Hames (1979) reported quantitative data upon the meat intake of a representative village of Yanomamö Amerindians located along a tributary for the Upper Orinoco River in Venezuela. Their observations extended through 13 months. They included a game-capture study of 216 days and a fish-capture study of 60 days. Sampling periods were designed to include all seasonal fluctuations in hunting and fishing opportunities. The measured intake was 75 g of protein per capita per day (adult standard) with hunting providing 50 g per day and the remaining 25 g derived from fishing. As noted by the authors, this was a minimum estimate since the data did not include meat eaten by hunters while on extended or overnight hunts, nor the protein resulting from casual consumption of insects (caterpillars, grubs, termites, ants, and bee larvae) and of freshwater crustaceans, frogs, and tadpoles by individuals of all ages.

In the absence of detailed information of the quantitative contribution to the diet provided by specific species of animals, as well as a lack of precise mineral content of tropical jungle animals, only a rough calculation can be made of dietary sodium gained from animal and fish consumption. If the United States Department of Agriculture's Composition of Foods (1975) is used as a source, the sodium content of 45 to 70 mg per 100 g of edible portions of various meats and fish could result in a daily intake of 2 or more mEq for Yanomamö ingesting 75 g of animal-derived protein. The contribution of unmeasured amounts of meat eaten away from the village plus various crustaceans and insects and the sodium intake associated with ingestion of cooking ashes represented additional but indeterminate quantities of dietary sodium.

One additional fact of life in a hunting and gathering society noted earlier must be emphysized. For the Yanomamö, as for many primitive hunting and gathering societies, life was a continuum of famine and feast. Hames (1980) has observed that on many occasions, male Yanomamö might travel in the jungle for two to three days with none of the band obtaining any animal or fish meat at all. These would be followed by days in which the calculated per capita intake of meat would approximate 400 g. Good (1987) also reported inconsistencies in successful hunts, with failure rates ranging from above 60% for hunts near the home area to less than 30% for those in remote sites. Even in times of plenty, sodium constituted a minimal dietary constituent. Thus, in this society, it appears that the physiological adjustments for handling of sodium must respond to a minimum intake of that ion on a chronic life-long basis. Evidence to support that premise for the Yanomamö has been gained from other studies which we conducted.

A second approach for estimating sodium consumption was applied in studies of representative Yanomamö Amerindians. Prior reports document that the measurement of 24-hour urinary excretion of sodium is a reliable index of minimum sodium intake in the absence of abnormal renal function or of significant non-renal losses from the gastrointestinal tract or skin (Dahl, 1958; Meneely, 1961; Joossens, 1971). This fact served as the keystone in our field work.

Biomedical studies of these Amerindians were made in a series of field trips conducted over two decades (Oliver, 1975; Oliver, 1981). Twenty-four hour urine collections were obtained from male Yanomanö Amerindians in four different villages (Figure III-11). Members of the expedition constituted control subjects. Urinary excretions of sodium and potassium are summarized in Table III-3. The urinary excretion of sodium averaged only 1.± 1.5 mEq per 24 hours, while excretion of sodium by the expeditionary controls paralleled values customarily obtained in acculturated societies. Potassium excretion was high in the Yanomamö and reflected the known high vegetable component of their diet. To determine that the finding of the extremely low sodium excretion was not an isolated phenomenon in the four selected villages, spot samples of urine were obtained from both male and female Yanomamö from an additional five villages at widely dispersed geographic sites in both Brazil and Venezuela (Figure III-11). For the 45 random urine samples obtained on the male subjects, the mean concentration of urinary sodium was 2± 4.8 mEq per liter; for 21 samples from women, the mean concentration of urinary sodium was 1±1.7 mEq per liter. Urinary concentrations of potassium were 107± 46 mEq per liter for males and 145± 63 mEq per liter for female subjects. In the overview, the accumulated data substantiated the Yanomamö Amerindian in the unacculturated state to be characterized as living in a "no-salt" culture.

Corroboration of our data on the Yanomamö has been presented (Carvalho, 1989). The observations reported 24-hour urinary excretions of electrolytes in 195 Yanomamö adults living in three villages on the Surucucu plateau in northern Brazil. Nearly equal numbers of males and females were represented. Mean urinary sodium excretion values were 0.9± 2.5 mEq / 24 hours and potassium values averaged 63± 32 mEq / 24 hours. The authors concluded that "when the sodium values are converted to salt, those individuals studied in the Yanamamö villages consumed virtually no salt". As anticipated from our earlier studies, systolic and diastolic blood pressures were exceedingly low, with a negative slope for systolic blood pressure with age.

For our studies of the hormonal adjustments to a lifelong paucity of dietary sodium, measurements were made of urinary aldosterone excretion and of plasma renin activity on samples obtained from one representative village (Oliver, 1975). The mean values for urinary aldosterone-18-glucuronide (Table III-4) were 74.52± 44.94 ± µg per 24 hours for the Indians and 2.7± 1.3 µg per 24 hours for the expeditionary controls. Similarly, plasma renin activity was elevated at 13.10± 14.17 ng per milliliter per hour for the Yanomamö in contrast to 4.94± 4.53 ng per milliliter per hour found in samples from the expeditionary controls (Table III-4). The values for the Indian subjects were similar to those observed for acculturated individuals studied after three to five days of a 10 mEq sodium diet (Oliver, 1964). In the overview, these findings suggested that the hormonal adjustments to a lifelong paucity of dietary sodium in the male Yanomamö resembled those found in acute sodium restriction of acculturated subjects and reflect a chronic augmentation of the major hormones responsible for retention of sodium.

Following completion of the initial hormonal studies in the male Yanomamö (Oliver, 1975), the impressive findings in that sample of subjects suggested that it would be of some interest to obtain similar studies in circumstances of physiological stress to sodium balance in this society. The two quite obvious situations are pregnancy and prolonged lactation. In pregnancy there are profound increases in maternal peripheral blood of renin substrate, renin concentration, renin activity, angiotensin, and angiotensinase (Weir, 1971; Skinner, 1972; Weinberger, 1976, Weir, 1976; Tapia, 1972). These changes are paralleled by increases in aldosterone secretion and excretion (Watanabe, 1963; Venning, 1956). In view of the estimate of an accumulative sodium retention of 500 to 700 mEq during normal pregnancy for the fetus, placenta, associated membranes, amniotic fluid, and growth of uterus and breasts (Gray, 1954; MacGillivnay, 1958), an augmentation of those hormones having a major influence upon sodium reabsorption is not unexpected. A further demand on sodium balance is the subsequent lactation which often extends over two to three years in this and other primitive societies and which occasions a daily loss of 3 to 7 mEq of sodium per liter of breast milk. These data obtained in studies of acculturated subjects served as the background for our investigation of the response of sodium-related hormones to the stresses of pregnancy and prolonged lactation in a sodium-poor environment. To control the possibility that findings in the Yanomamö were ethnic rather than dietary in origin, a comparison was made with similar studies of another Amerindian group, the Guaymi of Panama (Spielman, 1979) who, as described previously, have had free access to salt for a number of generations (Oliver, 1981). For these comparative studies, the field work with the Guaymi was conducted in 1975 and that with the Yanomamö in 1976.

In these studies, it was impractical to obtain 24-hour urine samples from the female subjects. Spot samples were obtained from the females between 8:00 and 10:00 a.m., while 24-hour urine samples were collected from the males to provide an assessment of total dietary sodium intake. For the Yanomamö, the subjects consisted of members of one of the same villages in which our prior studies had documented that the village had no access to salt (Tanis, 1973). Members of the expedition again served as controls for studies in the two populations. Isolated spot samples of urine were also obtained from the Yanomamö males and expeditionary controls prior to commencing collection of the 24-hour samples for comparison with similar samples collected from the females.

In the Yanomamö females, the concentration of sodium in spot samples of pregnant and nonpregnant subjects approximated 1 mEq per liter (Table III-5). In contrast, values were 119± 53 mEq per liter for the nonpregnant Guaymi and 79± 30 mEq per liter for the pregnant Guaymi. Concentrations of potassium were over 200 mEq per liter for pregnant and nonpregnant Yanomamö, but ranged from 106± 47 mEq per liter for the pregnant Guaymi to 138± 47 mEq per liter for the nonpregnant Guaymi.

There was no evidence of either hyponatremia or hyperkalemia for the Yanomamö, as serum sodium levels were 141.1± 4.1 mEq per liter and potassium levels were 5.3±0.5 mEq per liter. Values did not differ between male and female subjects. In breast milk samples from the Yanomamö, the concentration of sodium averaged 3 mEq per liter and potassium 8 mEq per liter. These are lower than the reported average values of 7 mEq per liter for sodium and 13 mEq per liter for potassium in samples from mothers in industrialized societies (Raye, 1977).

The most impressive findings in these comparative studies were the levels of plasma renin activity, serum aldosterone concentration, and urinary aldosterone excretion (Table III-5). Striking increases were observed for these parameters in the pregnant Yanomamö. For these subjects, the mean plasma renin activity was 25.6± 6.4 ng per milliliter per hour, the mean serum aldosterone level was 155.9± 245.3 ng per deciliter, and the mean urinary concentration of aldosterone was 585.3± 48.7 ng per milliliter. In contrast, concentrations of serum aldosterone were 85.5± 51.1 ng per deciliter in the pregnant Guaymi, while concentrations of urinary aldosterone were elevated to only 92.1± 110.1 ng per milliliter. Plasma renin activities were not measured in the Guaymi subjects. As expected from our prior studies, plasma renin activity, serum aldosterone concentration, and urinary aldosterone excretion were high in all the Yanomamö subjects, but those of the pregnant Yanomamö significantly exceeded values obtained in other members of the group. Despite the chronic sodium loss occasioned by prolonged lactation over a period of 2 to 3 years, it is of interest that the values for these two sodium-related hormones did not permit a distinction between the lactating and the nonlactating Yanomamö females.

These observations of the Yanomamö females provided the first data of the adjustments of sodium-related hormones to the stresses imposed by pregnancy and prolonged lactation in a "no-salt" culture. Other factors, both major and minor, may contribute to successful sodium homeostasis in this circumstance. These include the possibilities of an heightened appetite for substances of relatively greater salinity (Barelare, 1938; Denton, 1974) or temporary mobilization of skeletal sodium (Mitchell, 1976). We have no information about these factors. The ultimate fact is that the mothers and infants in this society appear to be healthy and with no evident disadvantage as a consequence of their customary sodium-poor diet. Reproductive success of the Yanomamö Amerindians, as reflected by a doubling of the number of villages and of greatly expanded hunting areas over the past 100 years (Neel, 1972), further emphasizes the absence of adverse effects of this dietary pattern.

A further insight into understanding the physiological adjustments supporting sodium balance in a "no-salt" culture has been provided by data on aldosterone binding serum proteins in some of these same Yanomamö Amerindians and additional subjects of this tribe from other villages (Nowaczynski, 1985). In parallel to the well-known serum proteins which bind corticosteroids, it has been established that serum proteins with a high degree of affinity and specificity for binding aldosterone are present in human sera (Nowaczynski, 1978a; Katayama, 1982). These particular serum proteins exist in thermolabile and thermostable forms.

For the study, samples were obtained from male Yanomamö and Guaymi Amerindians and from members of the expedition. By intent, pregnant individuals were excluded to avoid any alteration of serum protein concentration or activity related to the gravid state (Nowaczynski, 1978b). Binding capacities of thermolabile and thermostable serum globulins for aldosterone were elevated significantly in the Yanomamö subjects above those of the Guaymi Amerindians and the controls (Figures III-12a and III-12b) The elevations were present concurrently with significantly high serum aldosterone concentrations. In contrast, total serum corticosteroids and the binding capacities of corticosteroid-binding globulin were within the normal range for the Yanamamö suggesting a lack of dependence of the high aldosterone on stimulatory action of the anterior pituitary gland. These findings complement those of the renin-aldosterone axis in the no-salt society of the Yanomamö Amerindians. The simultaneously marked elevations of free, unbound serum aldosterone and of serum protein bound aldosterone suggested that secretion rate of the hormone was chronically very high in these people. That the high levels of aldosterone were physiologically effective was substantiated by the avid renal retention of sodium in the presence of a lifelong minimum intake of the ion. The data offer an additional dimension to the view of a group whose physiological responses have been keenly attuned to successful survival in a sodium poor environment.

The effect on health and reproduction occasioned by a lifelong paucity of dietary sodium must be considered from several perspectives. Although the Yanomamö Amerindians were semi-pygmoid with heights of the males at or slightly above 5 feet, they were muscularly built (Figure III-13) and displayed great physical stamina during their frequent day-long treks through highly irregular jungle terrain and at the tropical temperatures characteristic of equatorial latitudes. The Yanomamö sweat, but less than the expeditionary members who could not equal the strength or stamina of the Indians. Although measurements of sweat electrolytes were not obtained, the chronic hyperaldosteronism found in these subjects suggested that maximum sodium was conserved by sweat glands (Conn, 1949), as well as in the gastrointestinal tract (August, 1958). Other minimally acculturated groups living in low-salt environments had sweat sodium concentrations as low as 13.4 mEq per liter with potassium/sodium ratios of 1 to 1 (Macfarlane, 1970). It should be noted, however, that these subjects had mean urinary concentrations of sodium of 54 mEq per liter, obviously much higher than values found in the Yanomamö. Even higher mean values of 1.8 for potassium/sodium ratios were reported for another "no-salt" culture (Oomen, 1961). It is possible that sweat sodium values for the Yanamamö could be even less than 13 to 14 mEq per liter. In any event, it appears likely that the Yanomamö, who are chronically acclimatized to a low sodium intake, will have minimal loss of sodium through the skin despite obvious sweating.

In the course of our biomedical studies in over 36 Yanomamö villages throughout Brazil and Venezuela, we were impressed with the good general health of the mothers and the infants (Figure III-14). Despite the physical demands entailed in maintaining their gardens, often at quite a distance through the jungle from the village, and in the daily cutting and gathering of wood from the jungle for the nearly perpetually burning family fires, our physical examinations of over 200 Yanomamö women reassuringly suggested good general health. This was in the face of multiple stresses of prolonged lactation and superimposed multiple pregnancies. Simultaneously, the infants were well-nourished with no evidence of malnutrition. These findings must be considered in light of the recognized parasitic load chronically present in the adults and probably rapidly acquired in the infants and young children in an environment characterized by a lack of hygienic customs (Lawrence, 1980; Neel, 1975). In sites at or near sea level altitude, endemic falciparum malaria added an additional parasitic burden.

From 29 Yanomamö villages, detailed data regarding fertility, reproductive rates, and infant mortality were evaluated (Neel, 1975). Sterility was rare in the Yanomamö society, and in one observation of 40 women over 40 years of age only one failed to report any surviving children. Based on available information, Neel computed that the average

Yanomamö woman in the child-bearing age completed a pregnancy about every three to four years, with approximately 85 percent of these pregnancies terminating in a live-born child permitted to live. Again, based on available evidence, the average Yanomamö woman by the time of menopause had borne approximately 8.24 full-term infants, but because of infanticide or natural causes had a mean number of 3.20±1.5 surviving children.

The population growth rate of the Yanomamö has also been reviewed (Neel, 1975). On the basis of accumulated data, Neel calculated that the land area presently occupied by the Yanomamö was nearly 3 times greater than it was a century earlier (Neel, 1972). It was estimated that some 54 villages or village complexes existed within the geographic boundaries of the Yanomamö Amerindians of a century ago, while approximately 125-150 villages are thought to be distributed in the expanded land area of today. With the assumption that the core land area of a century ago had a village density similar to that observed currently, the calculated expansion of the number of villages per century would be by a factor of 2.3 times. Utilizing these estimates of expansion during the past century, average annual population growth rates were between 0.5 and 1 percent per year. Some data suggested that the annual rate would be as high as 2 percent (Chagnon, 1974). In any event, these calculations for the rate of population growth should be viewed from the additional perspective that this increase occurred despite the pressures of chronic tropical diseases and the high rate of homicide due to warfare (Chagnon, 1968; Chagnon, 1988; Neel, 1975).

For the Yanomamö, who constitute a genetically distinct tribe of South American natives, it is difficult to identify an overt disadvantage to a lifelong paucity of dietary sodium by the observations and biomedical studies that we have obtained. It is possible that other approaches investigating other aspects of the physiological adjustments to chronic low sodium intake by individuals in this or other "no-salt" cultures may reveal some abnormalities which can be associated with an adverse influence upon health, reproduction, or rate of population growth. However, the available information is quite persuasive that any findings of this variety are unlikely to document a significant negative effect of a lifelong extremely low sodium diet. For the individual male or female Yanomamö, general health does not appear to be adversely influenced, nor are fertility and effective rate of successful pregnancy reduced. Finally, the accumulated data documenting an expansion of the land area occupied by the Yanomamö, an over twofold increase in the number of villages identified in the total area occupied by this tribe, and an estimated average annual population growth rate of at least 0.5 to 1 percent per year suggest that, for this group at least, existence in a no-salt culture need not adversely affect the health of the individual male or female and the survival and expansion of the ethnic group.

In summary, reports and studies have identified tribes of South American natives living in no-salt cultures in the pre-Columbian period. Others most likely existed but their presence has not been identified by those early reports perused in the course of the literature search for this study. Perhaps of greater significance are the data describing the physiological adaptations associated with survival and successful expansion of population numbers in the Yanomamö society. These observations can be augmented by reports of somewhat comparable, but less comprehensive, studies of other groups.

TABLE III-1A: MINERAL AND NUTRIENT CONTENT OF REPRESENTATIVE FOODS IN THE DIET OF THE YANAMAMO AMERINDIANS*

	Ca++ mg/100g** Mean± SD	Na+ mg/100g Mean± SD	K+ mg/100g Mean± SD	Mg++ mg/100g Mean± SD
I. Garden Vegetables				
a. Plantain (n=4)#	3.55±1.2	2.2±0.2	345.09±83.5	24.22±2.6
b. Manoic, Sweet Potato (n=2)	48.71±10.0	4.88±3.1	347.20±35.9	37.71±3.0
c. Peach Palm (n=1)	22.4	1.6	216.9	22.4
2. Fish (n=4) (Piranha)	562.61±433.6	49.98±33.0	310.32±47.1	85.32±67.3
3. Meat (n=2) (Turkey, Turtle)	13.22±7.9	29.06±5.2	325.22±67.8	305.22±447.4
4. Eggs (n=1) (Turtle)	222.1	83.8	118.5	0.9

*Analyses kindly performed by the Analytical Chemistry Laboratories of the Gerber Products Company under the supervision of Dr. George A. Purvis, Director of Nutrition, and Dr. Sandra Pfieffer, Group Leader of the Analytical Chemistry Division.

** mg/100g of original sample.

#(n=x) sample size.

TABLE III-1B: MINERAL AND NUTRIENT CONTENT OF REPRESENTATIVE FOODS IN THE DIET OF THE YANAMAMO AMERINDIANS (CONTINUED)

	PO4 mg/100g Mean± SD	Cl- mg/100g Mean± SD	Protein g/100g Mean± SD	Fat g/100g Mean± SD	Carbohydrate g/100g Mean± SD
I. Garden Vegetables					
a. Plantain (n=4)	27.1±4.9	46.19±16.8	1.41±0.2	0.47±0.21	37.5±2.3
b. Manoic, Sweet Potato (n=2)	48.30±18.0	91.97±29.3	1.61±0.5	0.32±0.010	65.16±42.3
c. Peach Palm(n=1)	33.9	78.0	2.3	6.28	42.3
2. Fish (n=4) (Piranha)	536.36±310.6	84.33±48.8	19.40±0.7	3.21±0.92	3.75±2.7
3. Meat (n=2) (Turkey, Turtle)	186.59±50.2	55.04±18.5	18.71±4.8	1.21±0.26	2.21±1.0
4. Eggs (n=1) (Turtle)	370.8	144.8	12.2	8.55	1.4

III-2: MINERAL CONTENT OF COOKING ASHES AND TOBACCO PREPARED WITH ASHES BY THE YANAMAMO AMERINDIANS*

	Ca++ mg/100g** Mean± SD	Na+ mg/100g Mean± SD	K+ mg/100g Mean± SD	Mg++ mg/100g Mean± SD
1. Cooking Ashes (n=5)#	3408±1364	46±29	4676±2282	570±164
2. Tobacco (n=6) (prepared/unchewed)	3614±1933	24±8	3463±823	906±153

	PO4- mg/100g Mean± SD	Cl- mg/100g Mean± SD	Ash g/100g Mean± SD	Total Solids g/100g Mean± SD
1. Cooking Ashes (n=5)	659±558	91±63	62±32	125±21
2. Tobacco (n=6) (prepared/unchewed)	559±322	118±55	27±9	61±4

*Analyses kindly performed by the Analytical Chemistry Laboratories of the Gerber Products Company under the supervision of Dr. George A. Purvis, Director of Nutrition, and Dr. Sandra Pfieffer, Group Leader of the Analytical Chemistry Division.

** mg/100g of original sample

\# (n=x) sample size

TABLE III-3: TWENTY-FOUR HOUR URINARY EXCRETIONS OF SODIUM AND POTASSIUM IN MALE YANOMAMO AMERINDIANS AND CONTROL SUBJECTS

Subjects	Sodium Excretion mEq/24 hr (mean ± SD)	Potassium Excretion mEq/24 hr (mean±SD)
Yanamamö (N = 26)	1.02±1.51	152±74.51
Controls (N=8)	104.35±64.11	38.66±11.23

TABLE III-4: URINARY ALDOSTERONE EXCRETION AND PLASMA RENIN ACTIVITY IN MALE YANOMAMO AMERINDIANS AND CONTROL SUBJECTS

Subjects	Plasma Renin (ng/ml/hr) (mean ± SD)	Urinary Aldosterone Excretion (μg /24 hr) (mean±SD)
Yanamamö (N = 11)	13.10± 14.17	74.52± 44.94
Controls (N=3)	4.94± 4.53	2.7± 1.3

TABLE III-5: PHYSICAL CHARACTERISTICS AND RESULTS OF LABORATORY ANALYSES OF BLOOD AND SPOT URINE SAMPLES IN FEMALE GUAYMI AND YANAMAMO INDIANS.

Variables	Guaymi			
	Non-pregnant		Pregnant	
	n	Mean ± SD	n	Mean ± SD
Age (years)	9	25.0±4.7	7	21.6±3.1
Weight (kg)	9	55.6±7.6	7	58.1±7.8
Blood pressure (mm Hg)	9	113.6±7.9 74.9±9.4	7	114.6±7.1 69.7±8.1
Pulse (per min)				
Serum Aldosterone (ng/dl)	8	16.5±6.3	5	85.5±51.1
Plasma renin activity (ng/ml/hr)				
Urine				
Na+ (mEq/l)	9	119.0±52.7	7	77.8±30.0
K+ (mEq/l)	9	138.0±46.6	7	105.8±47.1
Na/K	9	1.0±0.6	7	0.9 ±0.8
Creat (mg/ml)	9	0.9±0.3	7	0.6±0.3
Ald (ng/ml)	9	7.5±5.5	7	92.1±110 @
Ald/Creat	9	8.3±5.7	7	128.2±97.2

From Oliver, WJ, Neel, JV, Grekin, RJ, et al (1981)with permission.

@This high standard deviation is due to one outling value of 330.

TABLE III-5: PHYSICAL CHARACTERISTICS AND RESULTS OF LABORATORY ANALYSES OF BLOOD AND SPOT URINE SAMPLES IN FEMALE GUAYMI AND YANAMAMO INDIANS(CONTINUED)

Yanamamö					
Nonpregnant nonlactating		Nonpregnant Lactating		Pregnant	
n	Mean ± SD	n	Mean ± SD	n	Mean ± SD
16	23.3±6.7	16	22.0±5.3	4	44.9±5.3
16	43.7±4.2	16	44.0±4.1	4	22.5±1.0
16	114.8±12.0	16	107.3±7.8	4	111.0±11.8
	71.0±6.4		67.0±5.7		72.0±9.8
16	85.1±17.0	16	83.0±11.7	4	98.0±9.5
16	47.8±59.3*	15	34.6±25.0	4	155.9±245.3#
14	6.2±4.1	16	5.0±2.6	4	25.6±6.4
16	1.4 ±3.0	16	0.8 ±0.7	4	0.7±0.4
16	215.6±86.8	16	264.7±71.4	4	262.0±66.6
16	0.007±0.013	16	0.003±0.002	4	0.003.±0.002
16	0.8±0.3	16	0.9±0.4	4	1.3±0.20
16	38.8±31.41	16	46.2±62.4**	4	585.3.±48.7
16	49.7±33.9	16	43.1±36.7	4	459.4±38.8

* This high SD is due to one outlying value of 256.

\# This high SD is due to one outlying value of 524.

** This high SD is due to one outlying value of 264.

South America

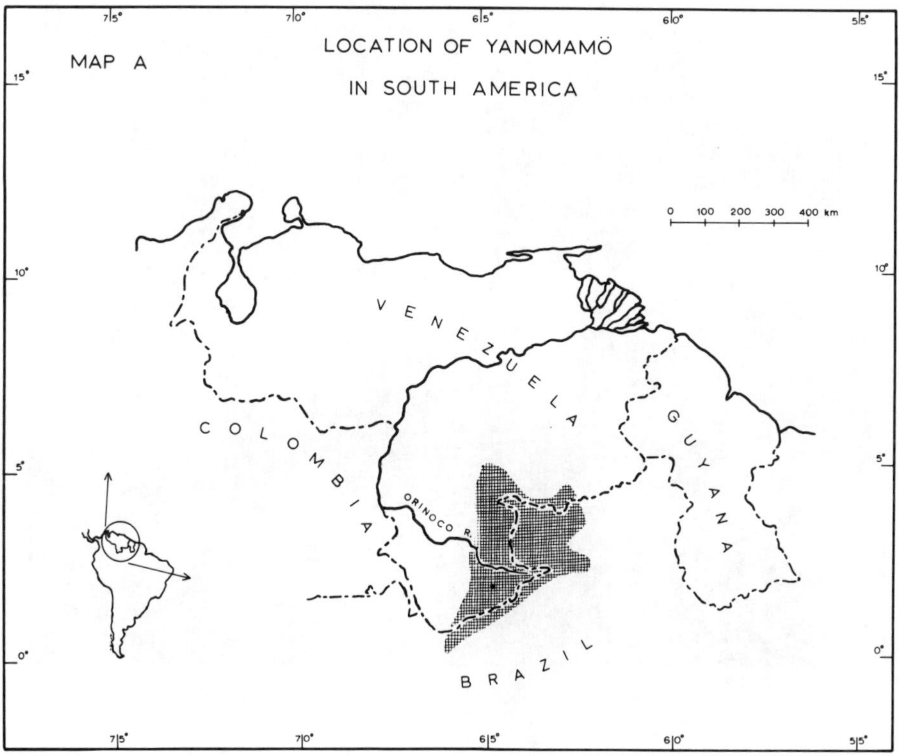

Figure III-1:Geographic distribution of the Yanomamö Amerindians in the interior of Brazil and Venezuela.

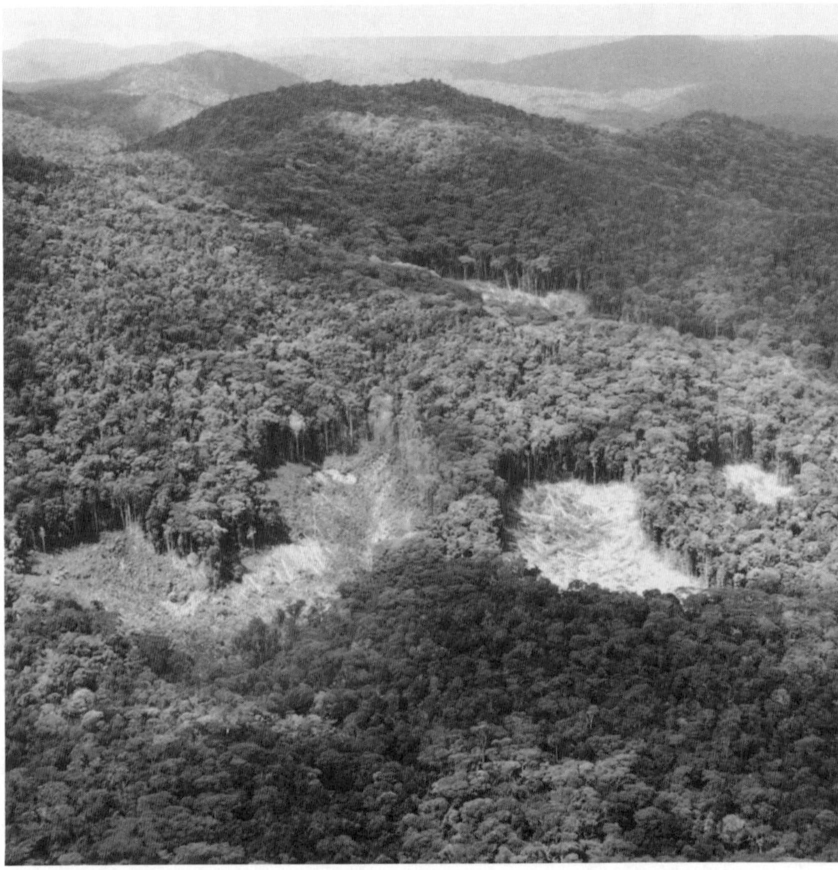

Figure III-2: Yanomamö gardens near the village of Marari, Brazil. A garden in production is on the left. The beginnings of two new gardens are represented by the dead trees not yet burned in the light colored patches to the right. A fourth garden can be seen in the distance.

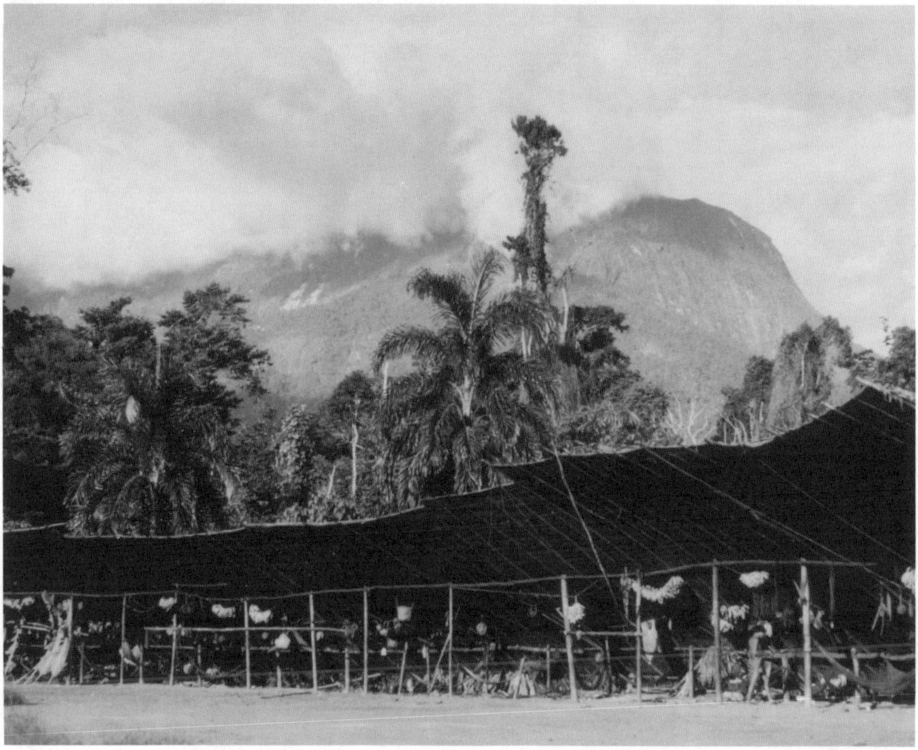

Figure III-3: An interior view of a community lodge, *shabono*, of the Marari village of northern Brazil. Numerous stalks of plantains (cooking bananas) are evident in nearly all of the individual family living areas.

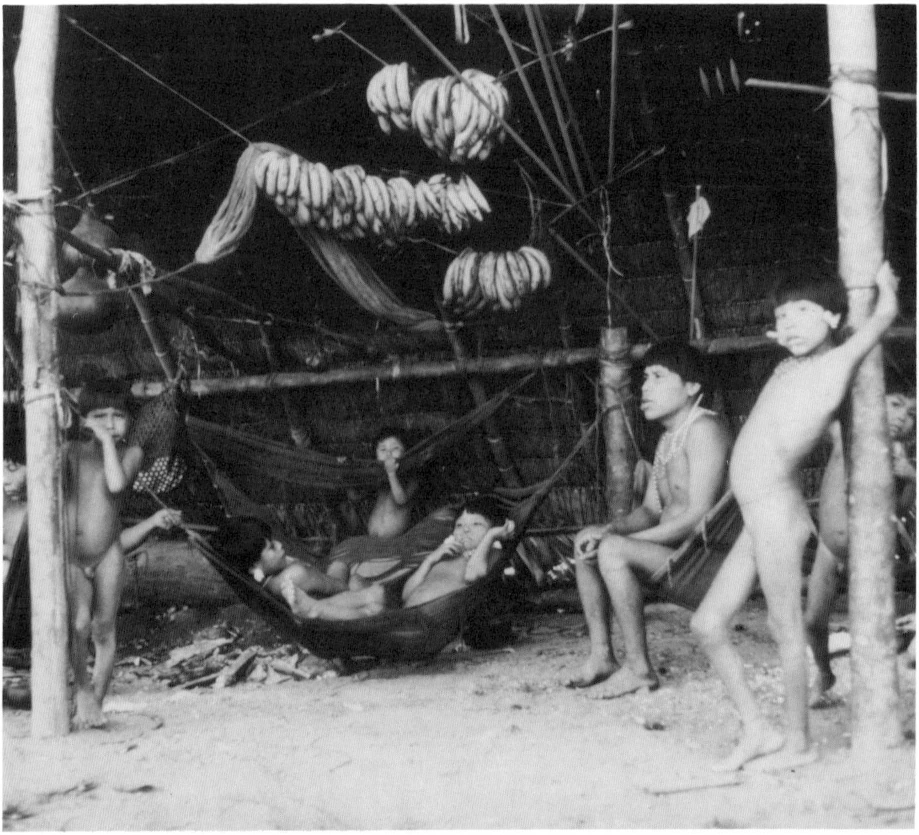

Figure III-4: A close-up view of a family living area. The plantains are prominent features in the photograph.

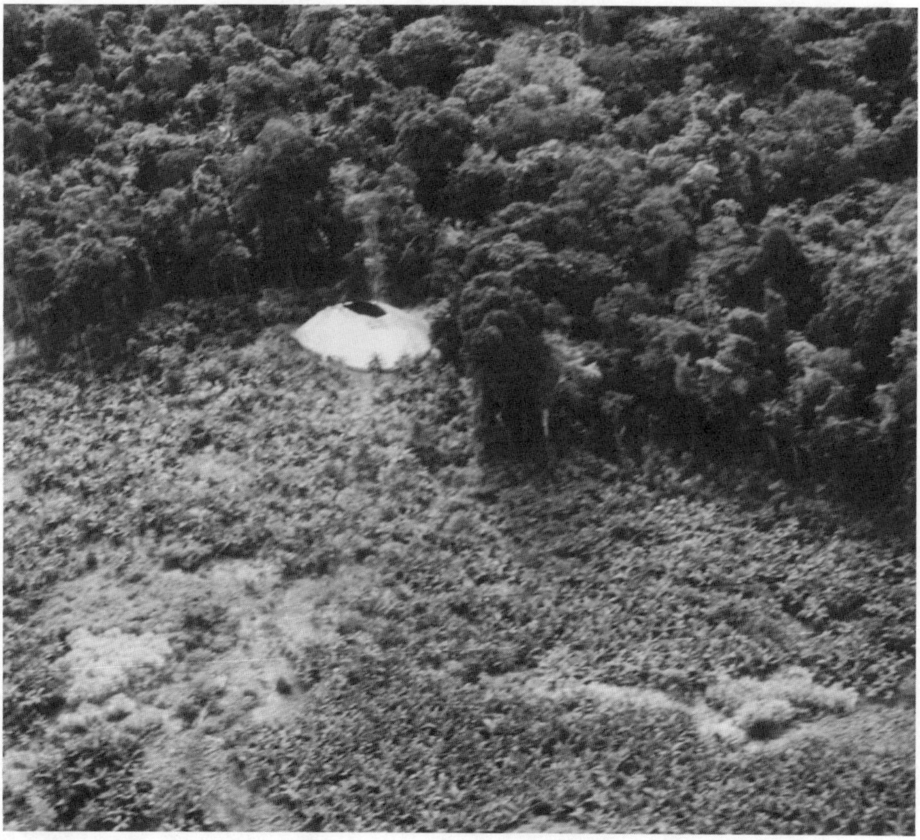

Figure III-5: A village community lodge in the Surucucu region of northern Brazil surrounded by a large garden with randomly mixed crops.

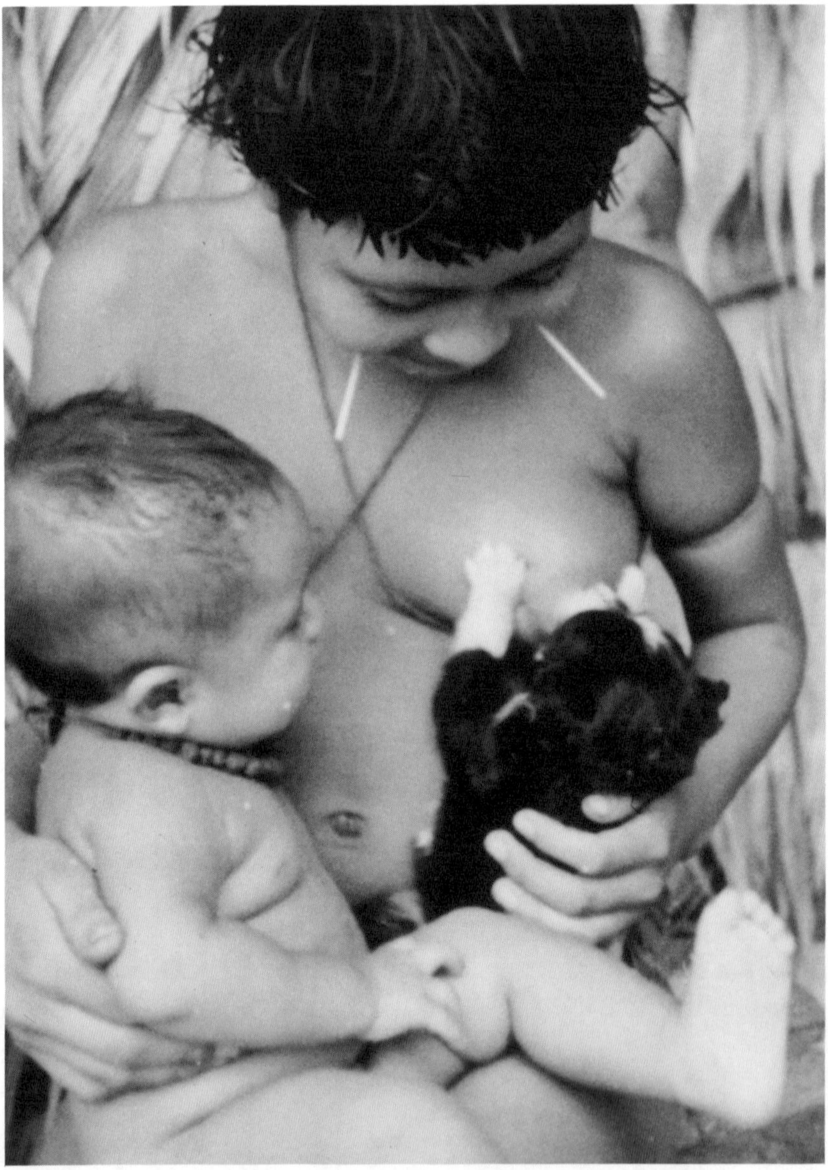

Figure III-6: Young Yanomamö mother breast feeding an orphan puppy.

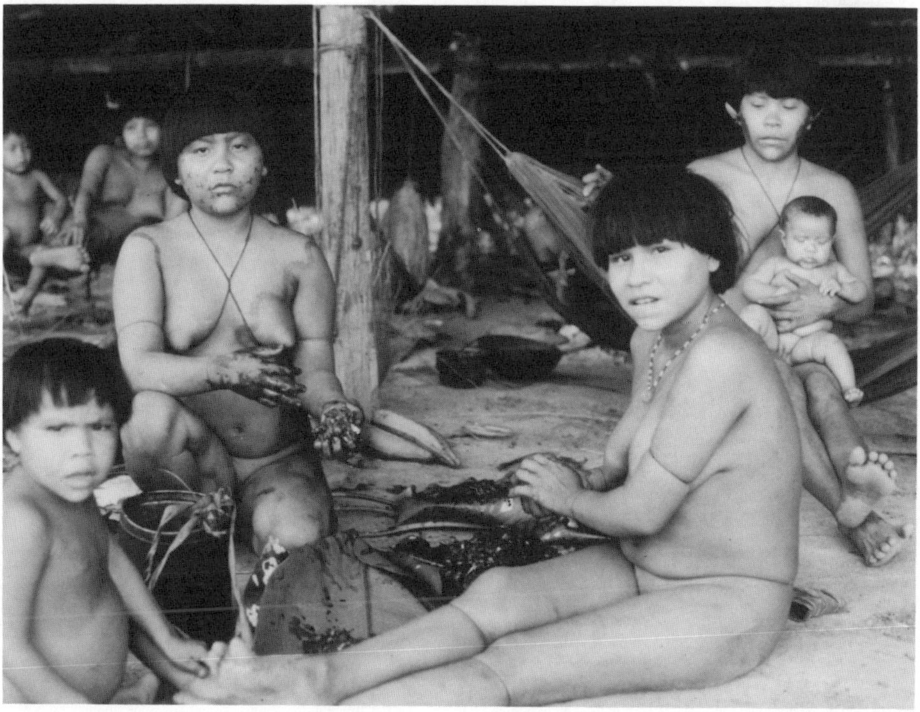

Figure III-7: Yanomamö women preparing caterpillars for the cooking pot.

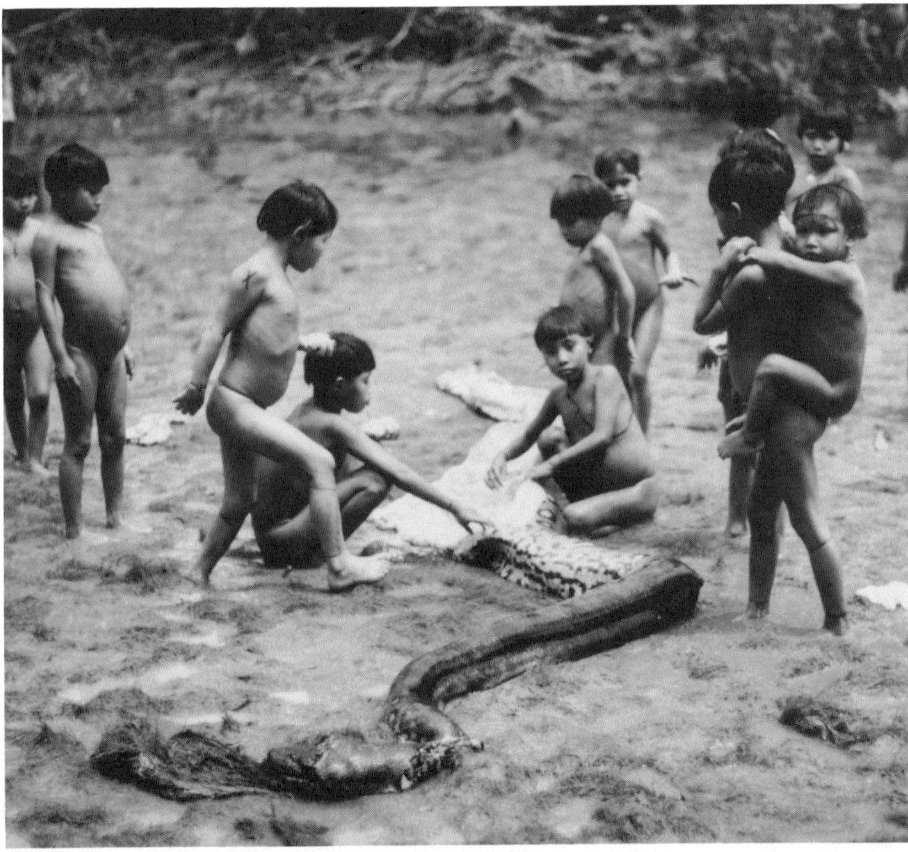

Figure III-8: Yanomamö children inspecting the partially butchered carcass of a 20-foot anaconda.

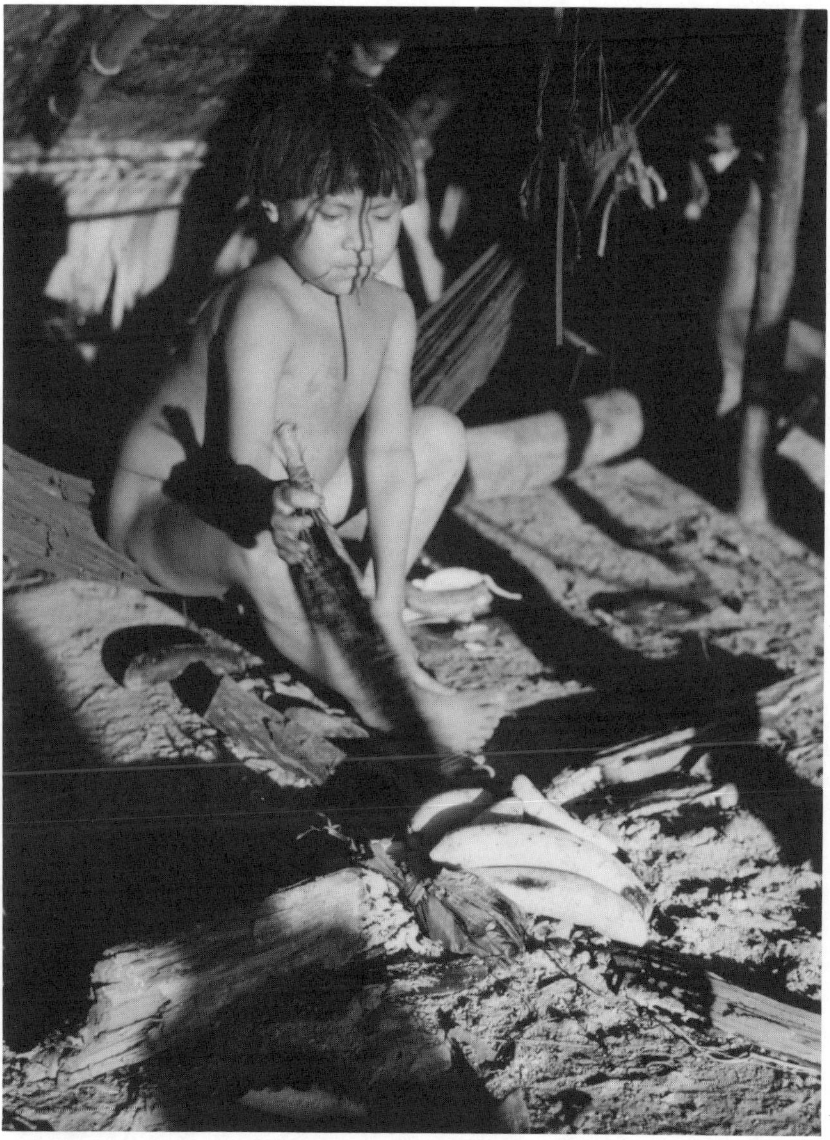

Figure III-9: Young Yanomamö girl roasting peeled plantains directly in hot ashes.

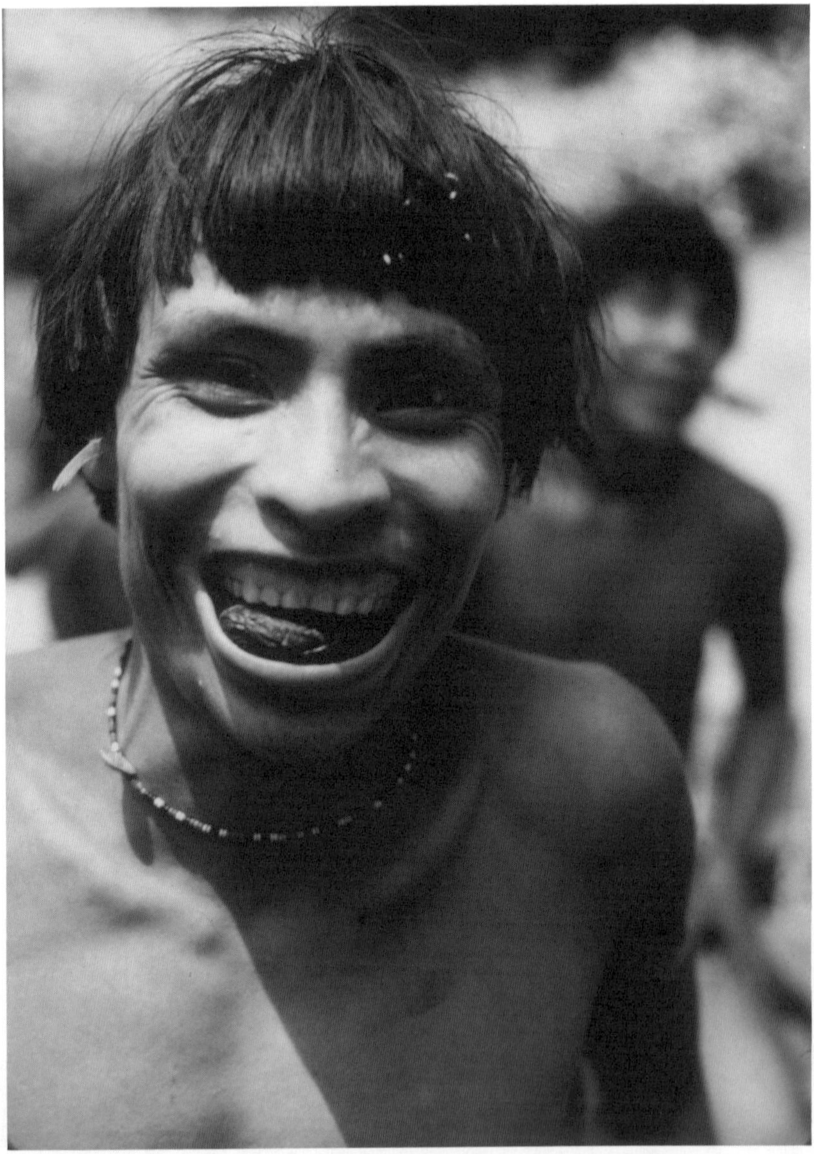

Figure III-10: A Yanomamö warrior with typical cud of green tobacco.

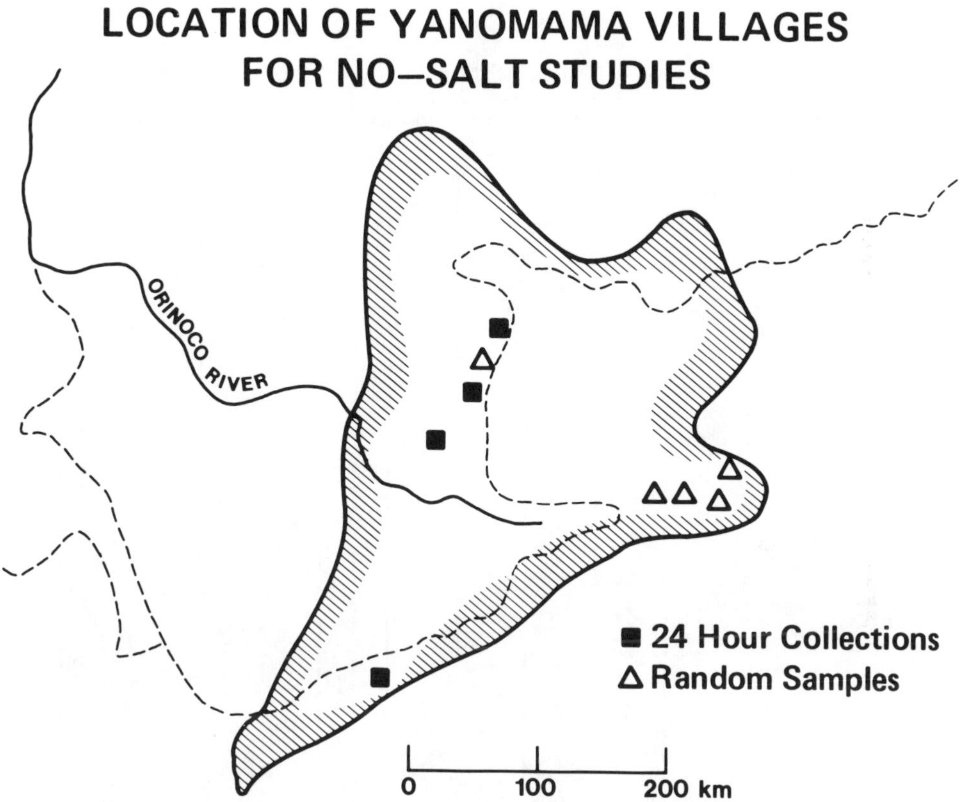

Figure III-11: Geographic distribution of the nine Yanomamö villages in which collections were made for urinary excretion of sodium and other elements.

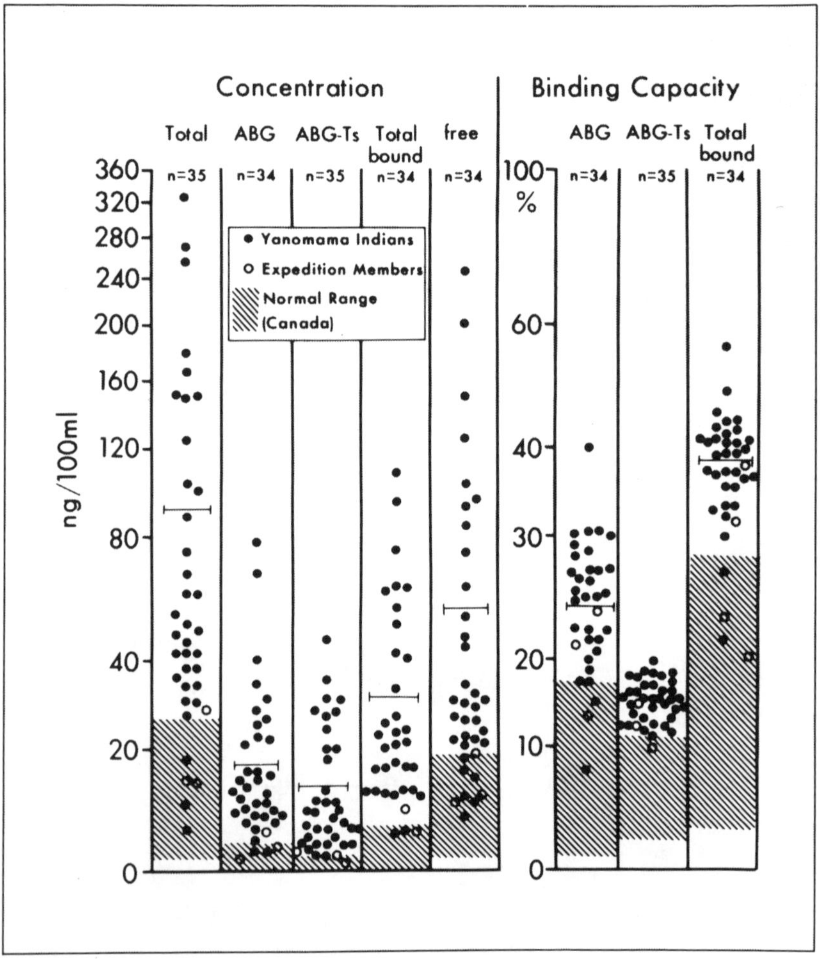

Figure III-12a: Serum aldosterone and serum protein-binding parameters in Yanomamö Amerindians.

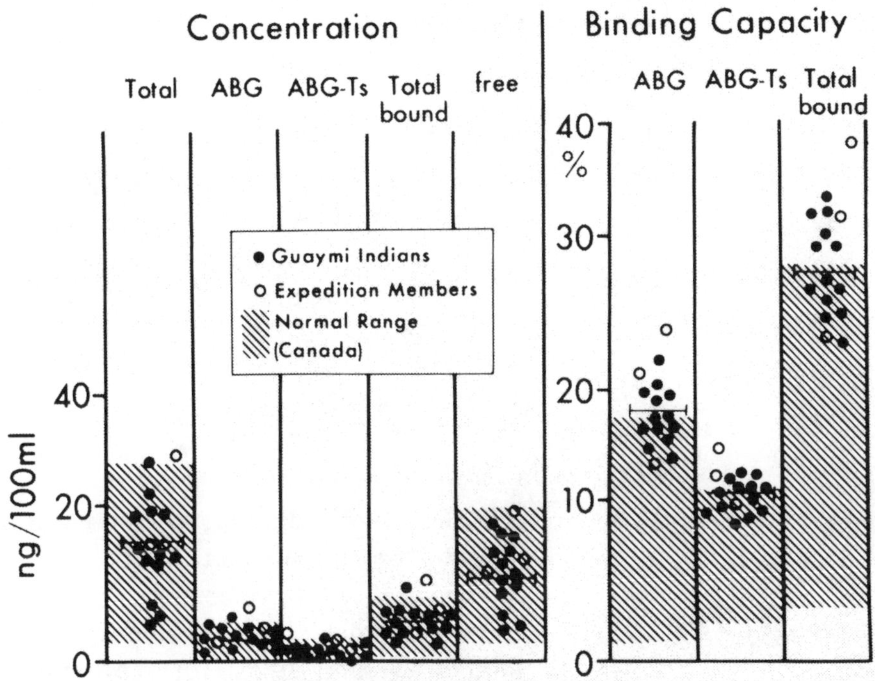

Figure III-12b: Serum aldosterone and serum protein-binding parameters in Guaymi Amerindians.

Legend for Figures III-12a and III-12b:

I. Concentration: Aldosterone.

Total: Total serum aldosterone.

ABG: Aldosterone binding globulin - thermolabile.

ABG-Ts: Aldosterone binding globulin - thermostabile.

Total bound: ABG plus ABG-Ts.

free unbound aldosterone.

II. Binding Capacity:

ABG: Per cent of thermolabile bound aldosterone relative to total serum aldosterone present.

ABG-Ts: Per cent of thermostable bound aldosterone relative to total serum aldosterone present.

Total bound: ABG plus ABG-Ts relative to total serum aldosterone.

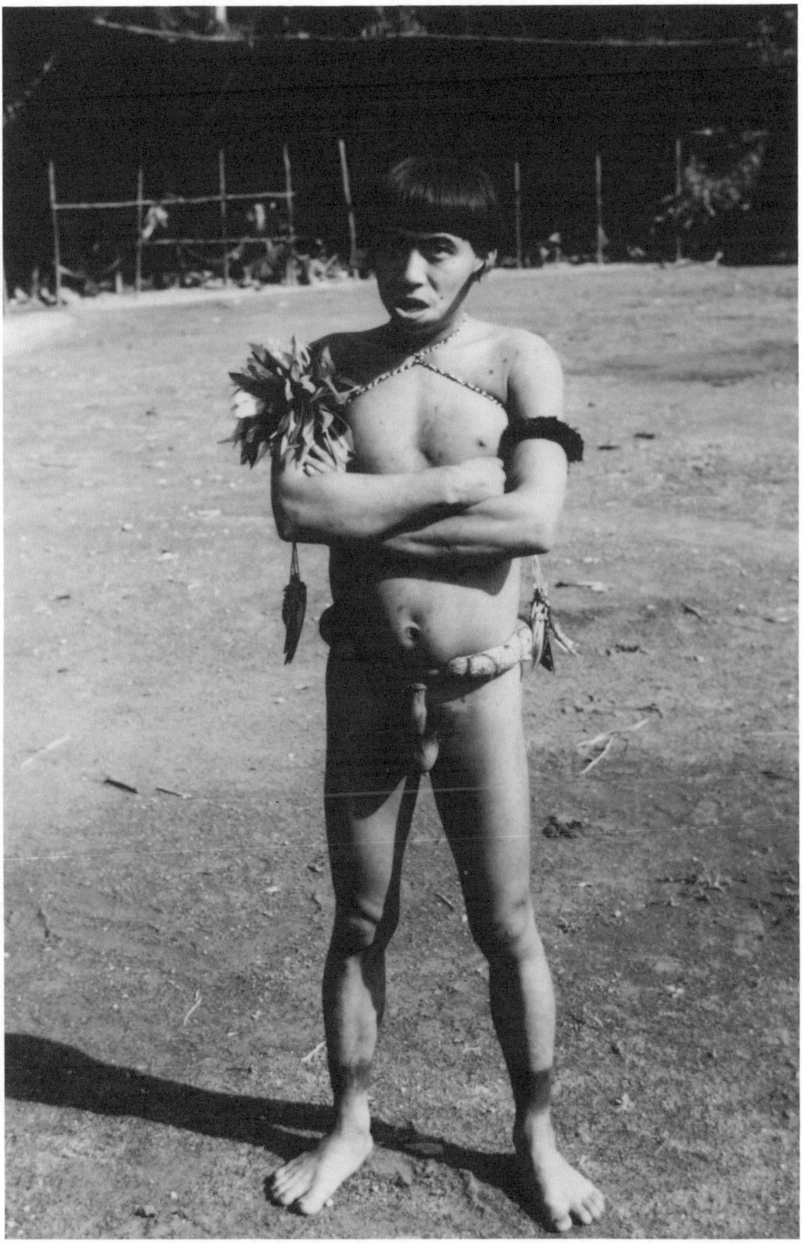

Figure III-13: A Yanomamö warrior.

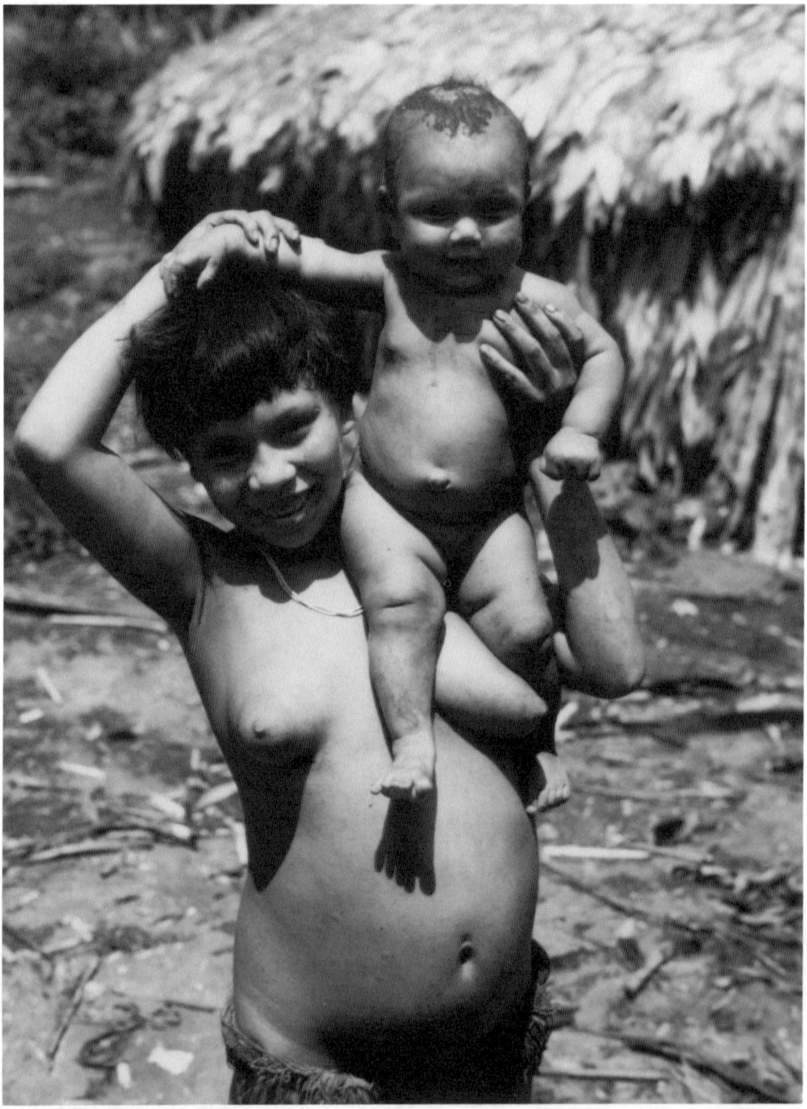

Figure III-14: A young Yanomamö mother and her infant.

South America

IV. Pacific Islands (Oceania)

Oceania consists of well over 20,000 islands scattered across the Pacific extending east to the Easter Islands, south to include New Zealand, north to Midway Island and the Mariana Islands, and west to include New Guinea. It is postulated that the inhabitants of Oceania migrated southward from Asia in multiple phases commencing several thousand years ago (Bellwood, 1980; Inder, 1977). The dispersion of the early migrants among different islands with relative isolation for many generations led to the emergence of the three major groups inhabiting the area. These are: the Melanesians occupying islands of the southwestern Pacific, north and east of Australia; the Micronesians occupying islands lying to the north in the region of the Pacific below Japan; and the Polynesians occupying islands with the widest geographic distribution ranging from New Zealand in the south to Midway Islands in the north and to Easter Island in the east. The appearance and anthropometric differences among these three races are associated with other distinct genetic differences as illustrated by the variation in tooth size and in frequency of the major blood groups (Brace, 1980; Simmons, 1966). It is to be emphasized that the Aborigines of Australia are thought to constitute an entirely different racial group from the inhabitants of Oceania.

The diet of the Pacific Island peoples was traditionally as varied as the topography of their island homes. For those living on the coast, fish and crustaceans served as a major source of protein, complemented by fruit of the breadfruit and pandanus trees and the meat of coconuts from the coconut palm. For those living inland, the range of comestibles included larvae, beetles, frogs, eels, fish, lizards, marsupials, and birds. Quite early following European contact, the domesticated pig was added to the menu of protein sources but often was eaten only on the occasion of a special celebration. Additional vegetable foods included numerous varieties of taro, sweet potatoes, plantains, and edible greens. Non-agricultural tribes, such as the Tuhoe of the north island of New Zealand, existed on wild vegetables and a limited protein intake (Best, 1902). For the majority of Pacific Ocean islanders, vegetables constituted the greatest bulk of the diet. Many of the diets, including the Maori, were observed to be deficient in protein and in the event of adverse climatic conditions, groups could be faced with near starvation until a change of seasons occurred with maturing of various plants, berries, and seeds and the return of migrant birds or spawning fish. Cannibalism was indigenous to a number of groups, including natives of the Solomon Islands, the Fore and Miyanmin of New Guinea, and the Maori of New Zealand (Alpers, 1965; Best 1902; Dornstreich, 1974). Determination of which humans were considered edible or taboo was associated with marked individuality of the various tribal groups.

Preparation and preservation of food similiarly varied widely. Obviously, many of the vegetable foods were eaten raw, while others, such as the potato, taro, and plantain were cooked. This was also true of the bread made from the heart of the sago palm and which served as a carbohydrate source for certain of the Melanesian groups. In most groups, women were responsible for the cooking, although men cooked for themselves when on the trail. Among the exceptions were the Mbotgate of Malekula Islands in the New Hebrides, where because of various taboos, the men usualy cooked for themselves while the women cooked for themselves and the children (Sorenson, 1973).

Food was often roasted on some form of spit above the fire or simply covered with hot ashes and coals. Many of the islanders used the steam oven, or *hangi*, which consisted of building a fire in a pit slightly more than one foot in depth with stones on the top of the fire. When the stones had become extremely hot, the embers were raked from the hole and the bottom lined with the then heated stones. Ferns were used to cover the stones, and the sides of the pit were lined with a woven mat or flax leaves. The food to be cooked, whether meat, birds, fish, tubers, or greens, was placed upon the ferns, which were then generously sprinkled with water and covered with several mats woven of flax leaves. The final step was a covering of dirt over the hole. Following a variable interval of time, dependent upon the type of food and the quantity, the coverings were removed and the food served. A combination of culinery experience and elements of chance dictated whether the meal was grossly overcooked or yet in the near raw state.

Among the peoples of Oceania, the use of salt or salt substitutes in the preparation of food constituted the full spectrum of possible variations. The lack of consistency, as will be evident in review of available data, occurred among groups living in nearly adjacent geographic proximity.

A. Maoris

The Maoris are the indigenous inhabitants of the New Zealand Islands. They are members of the Polynesian race and are thought to have immigrated in successive waves from islands northeast of New Zealand (Dansey, 1947). The timing of the initial immigration by the Maoris is not known for certain because Maoris had no written language, but Simmons (1976), following a comprehensive review of the available genealogies, concluded the information to be compatible with tentative dates for the first migrations to have occurred in the fourteenth century A.D. As noted by Best (1952): "The Maori language is a dialect of the far-spread Polynesian tongue spoken from New Zealand northward to the Hawaiian or Sandwich Islands and from Easter Island westward to Samoa."

The absence of salt in the Maori diet was observed by Brunner (1851) in his account of an expedition which he took to the interior of the South Island and on which he was accompanied by two Maori men and their wives. The duration of this walking expedition approached 550 days. In his journal he mentioned losing all of his salt in a heavy rain on the 150th day of the expedition without replenishment for the remainder of the trip. He subsequently noted that the preservation of eels by smoking by his native companions: "If properly prepared, will last some months." In describing the preservation of deboned birds, rats, and freshwater eels in airtight containers in their own extracted fat following cooking by application of red hot stones to the cleaned carcass, Brunner further observed: "I have tasted birds kept two years in this manner, and found them very good."

The most comprehensive reports of the customs and traditions of the primitive Maoris were compiled by Elsdon Best in a series of publications extending over a period of 30 years (Craig, 1964). As one of founders of the Journal of the Polynesian Society and a self-trained but highly disciplined ethnologist, Best detailed his observations of the Tuhoe tribe living in the mountainous, densely forested region of the Urewera country located in the north central interior of the North Island. To Best and his colleagues, the Tuhoe represented the last primitive Maori living in an unacculturated society in the late nineteenth century (Best, 1902; Best, 1925; Best, 1952). The area of their domain in the Ruatahuna Valley was located between the current city of Rotorua to the northwest and to Hawke Bay on the southeast. As observed by Best (1902):

"The natives lived in small, scattered settlements, each consisting of a few huts situated in a clearing."

The Tuhoe were a non-agricultural tribe, since the terrain was unsuited to agriculture. Thus, this group was compelled to subsist upon the products of forest and stream. It was not until the Europeans introduced the potato to the natives living in coastal areas that this plant was eventually traded inland and cultivated. A major staple of the indigenous diet was the fern-root (*aruhe*) which was obtained by use of a digging stick. Other staples included the roots of bullrushes, pollen of several plants, and the cabbage tree of which leaves, trunk, and root were considered edible. Berries covered with a mealy substance were used as the basis for a form of breadcake. Principal sources of animal protein consisted of the native birds, rats, freshwater eels and fish, and on special occasions, dog or human flesh. However, vegetables constituted the bulk of the diet.

For the Maori, the search for food occupied much of their thoughts, time, and skills. Preparation of the hard-sought vegetables was an additional burden of time and effort. The major staple, the fern-root, required drying before being beaten to separate the meal from inedible fiber. Cakes were made of the resultant meal and roasted in a fire. Similar effort was required for other vegetables.

In reference to protein, in his section entitled "Food Products of Tuhoeland," Best (1902) observed.:

"The Maori larder was sadly deficient in flesh foods, and this may possibly have had something to do with their cannibalism, for they were undoubtedly fond of human flesh as a food, with the exception of those who were *koto* -- i.e., who had a repugnance towards that unnatural diet.

"The domestic dog (*kuri*) was not numerous enough to form an important item in the native bill-of-fare, but its flesh was highly esteemed. This dish, however, only appeared on important occasions, as at a feast, or when prepared for a distinguished visitor. The hindquarters of the *kuri* are said to have been the best eating. Its flesh was sometimes used as an *o matenga*, or food for the death journey, on account of its delicacy from a Maori point of view. When a person was near unto death a special food would be prepared as a last meal for the dying person. Earthworms (*toke*) were a favourite article for this purpose, and it is said that the sweet flavour (*tawara*) of that prized food would be detected on the palate of the eater for two days after the meal.

"The flesh of the *kiore*, or the native rat, was highly prized by the Maori, and formed one of the principal food-supplies of Tuhoeland. This little creature was very numerous in this district formerly, more especially on the high-lying ranges, where it fed on the beech mast, and was trapped in great numbers. It disappeared about the early 'fifties.' This expression *'tau niho roa'* was applied to a season when the *kiore* were particularly numerous, and hence bold in stealing from the food-stores of the natives. The flesh of the rat was preserved for future use in the same manner that birds were -- viz., by taking out the bones and placing the flesh in a vessel, which was then filled up with melted fat, which preserved the contents. Rats and birds preserved in this manner are termed *huahua*. Old natives say that the bones of the rat were pulled out quite easily, that the flesh did not appear to adhere to them. When cooked for immediate consumption the rat was wrapped in leaves of the fern termed *petipeti* and placed in the *hapi*, or steam-oven. Such a wrapper or envelope for birds or fish is termed *kipaki* or *poutaka*. The rat was cooked without being skinned. They were caught in traps and pits, which we will describe later on. It is said that two kinds of rats obtained here, the *matapo*, a black variety, and the *tokoroa*, a grey one.

"Regarding the cannibalism of the Maori, human flesh was not only eaten after a battle, but also it was preserved for future use as *huahua*, in the manner described above. When rations fell short or some special food was required for a feast or to place before a guest a slave would be very likely knocked on the head, and his body consigned to the oven. Again, special raids were often made for the purpose of procuring human flesh or to capture a person to be slain, cooked, and eaten, in order to give prestige to certain rites of old, such as the opening of a new house, the tattooing of a chief's daughter, or the performance of the tua rite over a newborn child."

The Maori of the interior had no salt nor sources of substances of high salinity. In discussing the preparation of juice from the *tutu* berry, Best noted that properly prepared berries were quite harmless, but:

"If eaten before being strained, and so freed from the poisonous *huarua*, then the result is disastrous. Many natives died from eating these berries in former times, principally children. Persons so affected were placed bodily into cold water, and, it is said, would sometimes recover when treated so. Since the advent of the Europeans, salt has been used as an antidote for *tutu* poisoning; presumably it was used as an emetic."

Florence Harsant (1979) mentioned the use of salt by women of the Maori tribe of the Waitahanui village on the shores of Lake Taupo in the North Island in the early 1900's:

"The women (Maori) had been taught by the early missionaries to make leavened bread in their camp ovens, and apart from the fact that they never added salt, it was good eating."

On observing a long pit near her home Harsant commented:

"I asked the elders about it, and was told there was an old hangi or oven pit, where enemy warriors had been cooked after they were slain in battle. The length of the pit, which had puzzled me, was due to the fact that it had been customary at Waitahanui not to cut up the bodies as was normally done elsewhere, but to cook them whole. In 1905 those cannibal days were not too far distant in time, and there were indeed two old women in the *pa* who had eaten flesh. They told me *pakeha* (white) flesh was not as good as Maori because it was too salty! Certainly it is a fact that the Maoris, although fond of sea food, did not care for salt; it was never added to the food they cooked. The baker at Taupo did not salt his bread because the majority of his customers were Maoris."

Information concerning salt is available in the Maori dictionary prepared by Reed (1948) who stated that the Maori words for salt, sugar, Bible, tobacco, boot, Christmas, and tin are " . . . not true Maori, but are the Maori pronunciation and, therefore, the spelling of an English word which has become accepted usage."

From numerous sources, it would appear that the Maoris, at least those of the interior, did not use mineral salt. Coastal inhabitants who constructed storage baskets of seaweed for cooked mutton birds and portions of seals did get some salt from that source; however, since the cooked birds were coated with the extracted fat obtained during the cooking process, there may not have been very much salt. In any event, the inland inhabitants did not appear traditionally to have used salt or substances of high salinity.

B. Polynesians of the Small Islands of Oceania

Observations regarding dietary salt of Polynesians living on the numerous islands of Oceania were made only subsequent to intense contact with European culture. It is highly likely that native diets were grossly contaminated by customs and foods of the outsiders. Against this recognized background, the salt intake of Polynesians was the subject of two studies by Prior (1968, 1980).

Pacific Islands

In the 1968 study, a comparison was made between the natives of the coral atoll of Pukapuka in the northern Cook Islands and a similar ethnic group who had lived for 10 years or more in acculturated circumstances on Rarotonga in the southern Cook Islands. The former group had a subsistence level economy with a diet composed primarily of coconut, taro, and fish. The latter group had a cash economy with ready access to European foods including tinned goods.

Intake of salt was estimated from dietary information collected by the 24-hour recall method and by household dietary surveys. By dietary history, the Pukapukans only occasionally ate tinned meat and did not add salt to foods in cooking. In contrast, the Rarotongans consumed a considerable quantity of tinned beef and fish and used salted coconut sauce. Analyses of 48-hour collections of urine were made in a subsample of individuals from each of the two groups, plus analyses of casual samples of urine from most subjects. For the natives living in the less acculturated economy, the mean urinary sodium excretion was 63 mEq per 24 hours, while for the more acculturated group the mean urinary sodium excretion was 110 mEq per 24 hours. In this study, there was no significant correlation between the 24-hour sodium excretion and concentrations of sodium in casual samples obtained from the same subjects. The authors make no comment regarding significant differences in health of the two groups beyond noting that the subjects residing in Rarotonga were generally taller and heavier than those living in Pukapuka.

Prior's (1980) second investigation involved inhabitants of the three Tokelau Islands in the central Pacific area north of Western Samoa. At the time of the study, the Tokelauans were agriculturalists with their principal crops consisting of coconut (which was the most important), bread fruit, edible forms of pandanus, and pulaka (*Cytosperma chamissonis*). Main sources of protein were fish until the introduction of pigs and chickens following European contact. Pigs and chickens were eaten only on special occasions. Small amounts of flour, rice, and refined sugar were consumed, but dairy products were rarely in the diet. A multidisciplinary study of these peoples was conducted prospectively before their indigenous Polynesian culture had been eroded by significant European contact following migration to New Zealand. One facet included assessment of salt intake. The population of the three atolls at that time consisted of 948 individuals aged 15 years and older and 844 who were under 15 years of age.

For the study of salt intake, 24-hour urine samples were obtained from a total of 143 males and 173 females. The peak 24-hour urinary sodium excretion in the males was 51.5±7.7 mEq for the 25 to 34 year old group and lowest at 30.1±6.9 in 15 to 19 males. For the females, the highest 24-hour sodium excretion was 44±4.6 for the 35 to 44 year old group. The lowest values were in the 15-19 year old and 55-64 year old groups with quantities of 28.5±3.5 mEq. The authors commented that the usual daily sodium intake was estimated to be in the 40 to 50 mEq range during the period from 1968-1971 for these islanders on the basis of two or more collections in 53 percent of the subjects. These highest values which approximate an intake of under 1200 mg of sodium daily are only one-half of the maximum 'Daily Values' by the American Food and Drug Administration.

Of interest was the observation that preliminary analyses of casual urine samples of the Tokelauans following migration to New Zealand indicated that the urinary sodium concentrations were higher. The increases were clearly compatible with a greater use of salt and salt-containing foods. Thus, as has been noted (Page, 1979), proximity to the sea need not be consistently associated with a generous intake of salt. Other factors related to specific components of the diet may have a far greater influence on total daily salt consumption.

B. Melanesians

The Melanesian villagers inhabiting the tropical equatorial rain forest of the interior of Papua New Guinea constitute a population which was virtually unknown until after World War II. Geographically, the interior of the island is characterized by ubiquitous ridges rising as high as 9,500 feet and river gorges dropping to 1,000 feet (Sorenson, 1969). When first contacted, the villagers lived in small hamlets connected to one another by foot paths. Despite a wide diversity of languages (more than 700 have been identified in the eastern one-half of the island alone), subsistence sources and dietary patterns were generally quite similar.

In a study of nutrition, Oomen (1961) noted the high dependency of each group of villagers on a single staple food which might constitute 90 per cent or more of the caloric intake. Major staples identified included the sweet potato, taro, banana, and sago with selection for a particular village based on practical consideration of the species providing the best yield. Protein intake was often limited. Depending on the affluence of the group, animal sources included pigs and a spectrum of wild game comprising the cassowary, cuscus, tree-climbing kangaroo, wallaby, birds, pythons, rodents, plus an assortment of frogs, lizards, spiders, beetles, grasshoppers and grubs. Cannibalism which occurred in some groups, notably the Fore tribe of Kuru fame and the Miyanmin, provided an unusual source but a disputed quantitative contribution to the diet (Alpers, 1965; Dornstreich, 1974). Food was prepared by baking, roasting, smoking, cooking in leaf packets, or cooking on or between hot stones, the latter employing the technique of the stone-oven (Polynesian "*umu*") in a manner used throughout other parts of the Pacific (Oomen, 1961).

Sources, preparation, and composition of salt were reported in detail by McKee (1955). Three techniques for the preparation of salt (sodium chloride) or salt substitute were described. In the coastal regions, sea water was used or was evaporated to provide a dry product. By nature of the terrain, importation of the dry mineral was limited to a few miles inland. A second method of preparing salt for several inland groups was the production of salt from salt springs. This involved the soaking of wood in the salt water and then drying and burning the wood. Analyses of samples obtained in the mountainous regions from both eastern and western portions of Papua New Guinea indicated that these samples consisted primarily of sodium chloride with a mixture of impurities of the incompletely burned wood.

In those areas in which salt springs were lacking, plant ashes served as a source of a salt substitute. McKee described the tedious process in the preparation of this form of salt. At Azana in the Menyamya region of the Morobe district, a tall grass called *pit-pit (Saccarum sp.)* was grown in an area of approximately 15 acres. The grass was harvested at a height of eight feet, then burned with firewood. The minerals accumulated in the ashes were dissolved with water, and the resultant solution subsequently was converted to a dried product by heating over a fire stove constructed for that purpose. The final product was analyzed and found to contain no sodium chloride but principally potassium chloride with a small amount of potassium sulfate. McKee noted that analyses of a similar product made from the ashes of a fern also consisted primarily of potassium compounds.

Sorenson (1969) reported the preparation of a similar product from the ash of an indigenous reed or cane (*Coix gigantea*) by the Fore tribe. Different villages had varying recipes to produce salt of a particular taste by using ferns, herbs, staghorns, creepers, barks and some wild grasses with the ultimate evaporation of the minerals which had been extracted with water from the collected ashes. Cakes of these minerals constituted trade items between villages and were exchanged with non-salt making villages for bows and arrows, stone axes, smoking pipes, tobacco, and other items. This custom was disrupted shortly after contact. Alpers (1965) noted:

"Trade salt began to displace the native salt (*taiyo)* which had to be extracted from ashes of reeds, leaves, bark and wood by a laborious process and consists mainly of potassium and calcium salts."

The new salt was considered more palatable by the natives. Its position as a relatively cheap trade item led to its frequent use by incoming Europeans for barter in exchange for native foods and services (Sorenson, 1969). After introduction of Western commercial salt in the late 1940's in the villages of the North Fore and in the 1950's in the villages of the South Fore, production of native salt promptly declined and had ceased by 1959.

Chemical analyses of 13 samples of native-prepared salt from villages on Bougainville Island and in Papua New Guinea were made by Wills (1958) (Table IV-1). For the first seven villages, sources of raw material for preparation of salt were various inland plants and species of wood. For the interior villages of Deri and Wissel Lakes, saline springs provided the starting ingredient which was soaked in leaves or vines. These were dried and then burned to give a combination of ashes and salt. Various leaching and subsequent drying techniques were employed to produce salt of nonuniform purity. The remaining villages were in proximity to the coast. Sea water alone or diluted with fresh water was used by some groups in cooking. Granular salt was made by these coastal dwellers by boiling sea water to crystallization or burning driftwood or the stalks of a seaside swamp palm. The salt-laden ashes were then leached and the resultant saline solution boiled to crystallization.

As anticipated, the salt prepared from the burning of inland plants and wood resulted in an essentially sodium-free product with the content of sodium relative to potassium ranging from 0.001 to 0.012 per cent (Table IV-1). Use of saline springs or sea water resulted in products with the anticipated high sodium content. Wills' report of chemical analyses of native salt samples well complements the descriptions of salt manufacture by McKee (1955) and Sorenson (1969).

In a study of endemic goiter, Choufoer (1963) investigated two populations residing in the central highlands of western Papua New Guinea. The first group consisted of residents who lived in the Mulia Valley and among whom 80 per cent of the women and 35 per cent of the men had a goiter. The second group consisted of a closely related people living in Tiom, a goiter-free valley located on the headwaters of the Baliem River. In Mulia, sweet potatoes and their leaves served as the staple food with additions of corn and several recently introduced vegetables. The vegetable diet was only rarely supplemented by pork. The residents of Tiom had a vegetable-based and protein-poor diet similar to that observed in natives of the Mulia Valley. In the course of an assessment of nutrition among the two populations, 24 hour collections of urine were obtained and analyzed for nitrogen, sodium, and potassium. The excretion rates for sodium and potassium are summarized in Table IV-2. Choufoer noted:

"In Mulia subjects nitrogen excretion varied between 1.5 and 3.6 g. per day, which corresponds to a protein intake of 10 to 20 g. per day. The excretion of electrolytes indicates an almost saltless vegetable diet, usually about 1 mEq of sodium and 80 to 200 mEq of potassium. The much higher sodium excretion in a few subjects can be traced to payment in salt for services to the settlement. Much the same values were found in the subjects from Tiom though their nitrogen excretion seemed to be a little higher. It is very probably that a similar metabolic pattern occurs in most parts of the central highlands."

In a comprehensive review of the nutritional status of the natives inhabiting the western half of Papua New Guinea, Oomen (1961) described in detail the paucity of the salt in the diet:

"In the highlands, the intake of sodium is often strikingly small. This can be concluded from ash analyses of the menu, as well as from determinations in urine. It is very probable that the average highlander obtains 40-70 milligrams sodium chloride from his daily fare (less than one per cent of intakes considered normal). On the other hand, potassium intake is about 3-4 times the amount consumed under normal conditions. In the mineral distribution of the sweet potato, in 'bush-salts' and in urines of the highlanders K/Na rates of 200-300:1 are recurring values. Diets considered normal produce urine rates of about 1:2. The K/Na rate in blood serum appears to be normal, but analyses of urine and sweat produces very abnormal values. (Table IV-3).

"The absence of a regular NaCl-consumption is a drawback to preventive measures dependent on the use of salt. Of these, the prevention of goitre by iodized salt is perhaps the most important example but the same may be true for the use of medicated salt in the prophylaxis of malaria."

Ooman's finding of mean sweat potassium/sodium ratios of 1.8 in addition to the large urinary potassium/sodium ratios suggested that physiological adjustments to maintain sodium balance in these natives were maximally stimulated as described for the Yanomamö Indians (Oliver, 1975) and the Chimbu Melanesians (Macfarlane, 1970) (vide infra).

A second study by Oomen (1967) focused on urinary excretion of nitrogen compounds and electrolytes in a small group of Papuan New Guinean natives. The subjects were inhabitants of Mulia, a remote mountain village situated on steep slopes in the Upper Rouffaer Range in the Chimbu region. The subjects were characterized as "skilful stone age farmers" for whom the sweet potato dominated the diet. Analyses of varieties of tubers from the Chimbu district, but not the village of Mulia itself, showed a sodium content of 0.001 to 0.02 per cent in the oven-dry product. In view of the steep slopes on which they were grown, the heavy annual fainfall, and the high prevalence of goiter, Oomen concluded that the content of sodium would be quite similar in sweet potatoes from the Mulia slopes. Twenty-four hour urine collections were obtained from both male and female villagers. Pregnant and lactating females were excluded from the sample population. Results of the measurements of electrolyte excretion for 30 natives and 20 control subjects are tabulated in Table IV-4. Oomen commented:

"The excretion rates of sodium and chlorine were exceedingly low. In Mulia, an average excretion of 1.3-2.1 milliequivalent of sodium (i.e., 75-120 mg NaCl) per day can be considered normal. In the adult males an average of 6.8 mEq was found, but this figure masked two high values originating from persons who had had access to the resources of the local missionary household. In view of the mineral composition of the sweet potato, and the absence of imported salt, these low values caused no surprise.

"A peculiar aspect, however, in several of the 24-hour portions were the ultra-low values. Of a total of 63 samples, 27 showed a daily excretion of below one milliequivalent, 19 below 0.5, while in seven only 0.2-0.3 miliequivalent sodium could be demonstrated. This meant that in one litre urine sometimes only 5-8 mg NaCl were present. In one individual only such low values were noted on two successive days; the others showed considerable variation. The lowest Na/K rate noted was 1/630 (mEq.)."

In a comprehensive investigation of dietary intake and expenditure of energy by New Guineans, natives of a coastal area and of a highland area were studied (Hipsley, 1965). Natives of Kaporaka, a coastal village located 75 miles east of Port Moresby, lived in clusters of houses built on piles 10 to 15 feet above sea level at sites located 50 to 150 yards from shore. Canoes were required to reach the houses from the mainland. Gardens were located near the adjacent shore. Subsistence commodities included yams, sweet potatoes, bananas and fish. At the time of the study, European food goods (rice, canned meat, fish, and bread) were purchased occasionally by individual families at Kaporaka, but their greatest use was at celebrations of various kinds held within the village community.

The highland village of Pari was located on a steep-sided river valley about five miles in length. Houses and terraced gardens were interspersed opportunistically on narrow steplike plateaus on the 45° slope of the north valley wall. The uniformly 45° slope on the south wall required extensive terracing to permit gardening. Crops included sweet potatoes, bananas, taro, sugar cane, leafy green vegetables, and beans. In reference to food patterns, Hipsley commented:

"Luxury items in both areas are sugar cane, salt, and chickens."

"In past years, salt was an item that was eagerly sought, and long journeys were sometimes made to trade for it. As pointed out in Appendix III, this native salt was made from plant-ash and was mostly potassium carbonate (Wills, 1958). Salisbury (1962) mentions journeys for salt by the Siane to another highland area where it was obtained by evaporation from springs. This latter salt was probably sodium chloride

(Wills, 1958). The prestige value of salt has waned, however, as it has become more readily available."

To assess intake and excretion of water, nitrogen, sodium, and potassium, 24-hour urine collections were obtained from 14 adult male and female Kaporakans. Collections were obtained from an additional six lactating females. The volumes of collections averaged 334 ml in the first group of subjects and 187 ml in the lactating females. In the putative 24-hour urine collections of non-lactating natives, the mean urinary sodium excretion was 8 mEq and the mean urinary potassium excretion was 32 mEq (Table IV-5). Slightly lower values for both ions were found in the lactating females. In comparison, a single European male control excreted 120 mEq of sodium and 69 mEq of potassium per 24 hours. Data from highland natives were limited to reporting mean urinary sodium/potassium ratios of 0.22 in samples from 10 lactating females. These values were identical to those found in lactating coastal females. Hipsley stated:

"Sodium chloride consumption is difficult to estimate accurately, but it is obviously very low in both the highland and coastal groups studied by us. In the highland group, sodium chloride was used sometimes, but not regularly, in cooking, despite the fact that salt was available in most houses and the people were aware that further supplies were readily available from us. In the coastal group, even though the climate was hotter, and ample sources of salt were readily available, no use of salt (or salt water) in cooking was observed by us during the period of our study."

A remarkable aspect of these studies is the seeming paradox between a geographic proximity to the sea and the very low dietary intake of sodium (as reflected by urinary excretion of the ion). Although the excretion (and by inference, intake) of sodium of these natives was not as low as those of some

Melanesians previously discussed, the values were nevertheless impressively low. That such excretion rates were found in natives living literally on top of the ocean adds an additional perspective for reflection. Other reports have contained similar data and have emphasized the fact that proximity to the sea need not be equated with a high salt intake (Page, 1974). This may be true, but in accord with dietary practices of the particular group under consideration, it is not an inevitable sequence.

Concerning general appearance and health, Hipsley reported:

"The populations of both villages gave the impression of being healthy and happy, although protuberant abdomens and enlarged parotid glands were commonly seen in the Pari children; adults tended to have small fat accumulations with advancing age."

The stamina of males between the approximate ages of 18 to 45 years of the two locales was examined by the "Harvard Pack Test." Twenty-two subjects at Pari and eight at Kaporaka were tested by this approach. Difficulty in obtaining volunteers from the older men at Kaporaka resulted in a higher proportion of younger men. The mean "score" ± standard error for the Pari group was 73 ± 3.8, and in the Kaporaka group it was 89 ± 2.6. The authors believed it was not valid to compare scores between the two groups tested. In comparison, however, with standards published by Consolazio (1951), both scores were rated to be average-to-good. Hipsley also noted that results of tests conducted on 254 members of the RAAF stationed at Bougainville showed an average test score of 77 ± 0.639 (Macpherson, 1949). Hipsley concluded that the natives studied had "a very satisfactory degree of physical fitness". The small daily intake of salt was certainly not associated with a lack of physical vigor in the peoples.

Sinnett (1973) studied all members of the Murapin tribe centered in the hamlet of Tukisenta in the western highlands of Papua New Guinea. Their homesteads were scattered along the valleys of three rivers at an altitude of 6000 to 8500 feet. These natives were described as primitive horticulturalists and pig herders with a subsistence economy based almost entirely upon the sweet potato. A dietary survey was compiled on 90 subjects. The authors noted that sweet potatoes served as the almost exclusive source of carbohydrate and provided more than 90 per cent of the calories, while fat provided an estimated 3 per cent and protein intake averaged 25 gm per day for adults. Sinnett stated that the traditional dietary pattern had not been interrupted significantly by European contacts at the time of the investigation in 1966. At the time of the field studies from 1966 to 1968, however, the tribal community had had 16 years of continuous contact with Australian administrators and Europeans. Cash crops, as one index of sociocultural change, were reported by 40 to 78 per cent of the males surveyed. Both European-owned and native-owned tradestores were patronized by the villagers. Although Sinnett stated that the high cost of food items was a deterrent, no information on purchases of salt or of salt-preserved foods was given. In view of the rapid adaptation and appetite for salt of modern manufacture (Alpers, 1965; Wills, 1958), it is highly unlikely that salt or salt-preserved foods were consistently absent from the diet of the Murapin villagers. The 24-hour urinary excretion of sodium suggests that this is indeed the true situation. The author commented:

"Certainly the salt intake was low in this New Guinea population, probably averaging less than 1 g per day. The 24-hr urinary sodium excretion measured in 273 consecutive subjects gave mean values of 13.7 (S.D. ± 18.1) mEq for 135 females and 6.4 (S.D. ± 12.3) mEq for 138 males, which agree with previous reports (Hipsley, 1965; Whyte, 1958). Sweet potato has a very low content of sodium and 'native salt' prepared from wood ash is a potassium salt (Wills, 1958)."

Assessment of physical fitness was made with the "Harvard Pack Test" conducted in 152 consecutive nonpregnant subjects (Table IV-6). Sinnett concluded that "good" or "superior" scores were gained by 76 percent of men and 36 percent of women. These results were interpreted to compare favorably with those recorded for other New Guinean natives (Hipsley, 1965) and British Commonwealth Divisions serving in Korea (Adam, 1955) but to be superior to those of Royal Australian Air Force personnel (Macpherson, 1949).

Macfarlane and colleagues (Denton, 1969; Macfarlane, 1970; Scoggins, 1980) have reported measurements of mean urinary electrolytes in the Chimbu tribe of whom the most isolated and unacculturated were the Tsenda, living in the uplands of the Jimi River north of Mount Hagen in Papua New Guinea. This primitive group had had missionary contact for three years at the time of the observations commencing in 1966. They practised a subsistence economy strategy with the sweet potato serving as the principal source of carbohydrate and calories. The authors described this tribe as existing on a vegetarian diet prior to contact. At the time of the study, Macfarlane noted that a mission had been flying in canned meat and the salt consumption had increased threefold since 1965 but was still considered low.

The mean concentrations of urinary sodium were 27 mEq per liter with associated potassium concentrations of 224 mEq per liter, yielding a sodium/potassium ratio of 0.12. In contrast, in the most acculturated members of the tribe who worked in Goroka as hospital orderlies consuming European types of food, the sodium/potassium ratios were 2.96 and approximated those of European controls. For members of the Tsenda tribe living upon a primarily vegetable diet, salivary and sweat electrolytes showed low sodium/potassium ratios in contrast to the acculturated native subjects' values which approached those of

European controls. Blood aldosterone concentration demonstrated a reciprocal relationship with urinary sodium/potassium ratios: the highest mean value of 23.2 ng per deciliter was found in the most unacculturated group. In the contrasting group who had had access to salt and tinned meat over a number of years, the mean concentration of blood aldosterone was 9.9 ng per deciliter. Despite the differences in salt intake and in blood aldosterone concentration between the most unacculturated and those in various stages of acculturation, plasma renin activities were elevated in all native subjects studied as compared with European controls.

In an investigation of blood pressure in Melanesians, Maddocks (1967) conducted a study of 50 individuals from each of 20 sites of the Papuan New Guinea Island (9). Among inhabitants of the 20 sites, the diets were based on a dominant starch staple which varied among the sweet potato, sago, taro, yam, banana, and rice in the different villages with little vegetable protein and scant animal protein. In a pattern similar to the observations of Macfarlane, acculturation was associated with increased salt intake. The mean ratio of potassium/sodium in the urine of 24 natives of the most unacculturated group of the Chimbu tribe was 24.2, while the ratio was 1.9 in the urine of 10 Hanuabadan tribesmen with an observed high intake of tinned food.

Additional investigations of salt intake have been reported for Melanesians inhabiting other islands. In a combined ethnographic, anthropometric, and medical study, data were reported for six distinct tribal groups of Melanesians living in rural villages in the Solomon Islands (Page, 1974). In this multifaceted study, cultural, demographic, and physical data were used to estimate the level of acculturation.

The most acculturated group, the Nasioi, had had continuous contact with European life-style and trade goods for over 80 years. Their economy consisted predominantly of settled agriculture based on several cash crops suplemented by the men working intermittently for cash wages. The dietary staple of this tribe was the sweet potato augmented by purchased tinned meat, fish, rice, and bread. Salt was used regularly in cooking. On festive occasions the diet was supplemented with pigs and chickens. The least acculturated group, the Kwio, were agriculturists whose diet consisted of 85 per cent sweet potato supplemented by leafy vegetables with grubs, insects, and freshwater prawns used as relishes. Pigs were eaten only on ceremonial occasions and principally by the men. Salt was also used on rare ceremonial occasions. In a poll of 28 Kwio men who were asked when they had last eaten salt, the responses ranged from one week to one year with a median of 18 weeks. European food was unavailable. The remaining four groups were between the two described tribes regarding acculturation.

In this study, salt intake was based on observations of dietary habits over a period of 18 to 24 months by the cultural anthropologist assigned to each of the six villages. Data of trade store inventories were obtained and sales of salt and salt-containing foods were monitored over a six-month period. These data were supplemented by personal interviews in which inquiries were made regarding the use of salt. Random urine samples were collected for measurements for sodium, potassium, and creatinine, but only a few were obtained in the less acculturated groups. Calculations based on all available data gave estimates of daily sodium intake for the more acculturated groups to range between 50 and 230 mEq per 24 hours and to less than 20 mEq per 24 hours for the most unacculturated group, the Kwaio. The group with the highest estimated sodium intake of 150 to 230 mEq per 24 hours were the Lau who customarily cooked vegetables in seawater. The authors reported that nutrition, physique, and physical fitness appeared to be good in all six of the studied groups.

Another report of interest concerning intake of salt by Melanesians is the observation by Wheatcroft (1973) of the Tifalmin tribe inhabiting the area just east of the Star Mountains in the interior of Papua New Guinea. Subsistence was dependent on primitive agriculture with the cultivation of many varieties of taro, sweet potatoes, bananas, and sugar cane. Animal sources of protein included spiders, tadpoles, lizards, toads, birds, rats, indigenous marsupials, and an occasional domesticated or wild pig. Because of strict taboos, women and children were excluded from many animal sources of protein. Wheatcroft noted that most of the tribes in the Tifalmin inhabited area did not traditionally use salt (Wheatcroft, 1974). They did burn a particular leaf which was sometimes sprinkled on food and most probably represented a potassium salt An interesting Tifalmin habit, which may have contributed to the intake of sodium and other minerals, was the drinking of opossum urine after they killed the animal.

For representative Melanesian groups, the observations and specific analyses of urine and other body fluids have substantiated a lack of use of sodium salt in the indigenous diet for many of the tribes. Promptly, with commencing acculturation, salt and food sources of high salinity were acquired by trade. The intake of salt paralleled to a remarkable degree the level of acculturation. Natives inhabiting coastal areas presented a diametrical contrast since some used seawater and salt manufactured from seawater in their diet, while others totally abstained from using seawater or salt derived from it. This paradox of similar ethnic groups in the unacculturated state being salt users or no-salt users is a recurring theme as the world is surveyed.

In summary, many of the inhabitants of the Pacific Islands were clearly living in salt-free societies at time of first contact by explorers and other representatives of industrialized societies. Simultaneously, the exceptions which are readily evident in the reports of groups seeking saline springs and sea-water for their sodium salt content emphysize the potential confusion that can confront investigators of native diets.

TABLE IV-1. SODIUM AND POTASSIUM CONTENT OF NATIVE SALT SAMPLES OBTAINED FROM BOUGAINVILLE ISLAND AND PAPUA NEW GUINEA*

Sources of samples (Villages or sub-district)	Na+ mg/100g	K+ mg/100
1. Guava	290	23,700
2. Onovi	250	26,850
3. Mumeng	112	45,500
4. Menyhamya	110	44,300
5. Droringgam	160	27,400
6. Amaiva	60	46,150
7. Chimbu	90	49,600
8. Deri	30,000	6,000
9. Mouth of Ramu River	7675	630
10. Mouth of Ramu River	9,880	4,820
11.Gwiarak	20,300	930
12. But	32,800	320
13. Wissel Lakes	29,500	218

*Modified from Wills (1958), with permission.

IV-2. INDICES OF NUTRITION IN SUBJECTS FROM MULIA AND TIOM*

Subject			Urine, daily excretion of [a]		
No.	Sex	Age	N (g)	Na+ (mEq)	K+ (mEq)
Mulia[b]					
2	f	16	2.3	1.2	182
3	f	16	2.2	1.6	190
4	f	25	3.2	1.2	174
5	f	35	2.3	0.5	148
20	m	16	1.5	0.5	84
21	m	17	3.6	0.2,25[c]	172
22	m	30	3.3	0.5	225
23	m	25	2.2	1.4	136
25	m	30	1.8	1.5	68
Mulia, houseboys					
78	m	17	3.2	4.0	81
79	m	15	6.8	61.3	121
Tiom					
202	f	20	3.9	0.9	222
203	f	25	1.9	0.6	117
204	f	25	3.1	0.7	209
206	m	21	5.5	0.7	205
207	m	25	3.0	0.7	285
219	m	15	3.0	0.8	236

a. In the subjects from Mulia the average values of 2 consecutive 24-hr urine samples are given; in those from Tiom the values obtained in a single 24-hr specimen.
b. For the analyses in this table well-developed subjects were selected, of adult or nearly adult age.
c. Separate values of 2 consecutive 24-hr urines.

* From Choufoer (1963), with permission.

Table IV-3. ELECTROLYTES IN SWEAT, URINE AND BLOOD OF HIGHLAND PAPUANS*

	Sweat	Urine	Serum (meq.L)		
	K/Na	K/Na	K+	Na+	Cl-
Local diet †, mean	1.8	216	4.1	142	92
Local diet †, range	1.1-2.8	9-105.	3.6-4.6	139-146	84-99
Local control ††	0.2	2.1	---	138	98
Normal values †††	---	0.6-0.8	3.6-6.2	135-153	98-108

† Nine adult male highland Papuans.
†† One male Papuan nurse, food partly imported.
††† Sunderman, FW and Boerner, F (1949): *Normal Values in Clinical Medicine*, Saunders, Philadelphia.

* From Oomen (1961), with permission.

Table IV-4. ELECTROLYTE EXCRETION IN SWEET POTATO EATERS AND IN EUROPEAN CONTROLS*

Subjects	Sodium	Potassium	Chlorine
	(Average per day in millequivalents)		
Highland groups:			
10 adolescent males	1.7	105	4.7
7 adult males†	6.8	180	4.0
6 adolescent females	1.3	123	3.7
7 adult females	2.1	138	4.1
Control groups			
10 adult males	177	49	174.0
10 adult females	154	55	149.0

† Two had some imported salt.

* From Oomen (1967), with permission.

Table IV-5. 24-HOUR URINARY EXCRETION OF SODIUM AND POTASSIUM IN ADULT KAPORAKANS*

Name	Sex	Sodium mEq /day	Potassium mEq /day	Ratio Na/K /day
Normal adults				
Kila Vali	M	2	40	0.05
Mulina	M	3	16	0.19
Mari	M	35	61	0.57
Kila Kopi	M	1	8	0.12
Kila Wui	M	18	36	0.50
Mula	M	8	40	0.20
Vavine	M	5	20	0.25
Kema	F	7	15	0.47
John Karo	M	2	68	0.03
John Karo	M	4	29	0.14
Kila Kila	M	1	14	0.07
Ren Age	F	22	14	0.16
Pala karo	M	5	50	0.10
Pala karo	M	1	42	0.02
MEAN: (14)		8	32	0.20
Lactating women:				
Kila Kipi		11	46	0.24
Mari-Aoneke		7	20	0.35
Laego-Guma		7	19	0.37
Manu		3	55	0.06
Kopi-Kwamala		7	37	0.19
Mala-Aoeneke		1	7	0.14
MEAN: (6)		6	31	0.22
European (living in New Guinea for 5 months)	M	120	69	1.74

* Modified from Hipsley (1965), with permission.

Table IV-6. PHYSICAL FITNESS: HARVARD PACK TEST SCORES*

Age Group	Males #	Males Mean	Males S.D.	Females #	Females Mean	Females S.D.
15-24	34	81.2	10.9	24	69.9	14.9
25-34	29	82.6	10.0	21	73.0	15.0
35-44	19	85.2	14.5	14	74.4	13.8
45-54	7	85.4	17.6	4	50.2	9.1
Total	89	82.8	12.2	63	70.0	15.4

* From Sinnett (1973), with permission.

V. Australia:

By the use of radiocarbon dating technology, the southeastern portion of the continent of Australia was shown to have been discovered by man over 30,000 years ago (Wright, 1977). Archaeological studies established an age of 32,000 years for stone tools of early hunter-gatherers at Lake Mungo in western New South Wales, and human bones from cremated burials were dated at 25,000 years by radiocarbon technique (MacIntosh, 1977). To date, however, it has not been possible by archaeological research to satisfactorily link these earlier occupants with the contemporary Aborigine. Available data suggest that the ancestors of the Aborigine can be traced back culturally and physically at least 10,000 years (Wright, 1977). Regardless of the present ambiguity concerning the progenitors of the Aborigine, it is the consensus that relatives of the present-day Australian native crossed to Australia from a more northern region during the late Pleistocene (Clark, 1969). At that time, sea levels were as much as 100 meters lower than today as a consequence of the last great glaciation. In the absence of geological evidence of a land-bridge joining Australia to more northerly land masses in that period, it is currently presumed that the ancestors of early man in Australia had to negotiate the open sea to reach that continent (MacIntosh, 1977). It is postulated that after landing at some northern point on the coast of the continent, the progeny of the settlers gradually spread over many centuries to all parts of Australia. Calculations made since 1788 suggested that at the time of the first European contact the total Aborigine population of Australia approximated 300,000 (Elkin, 1964).

Evidence obtained by blood group and serum protein gene frequencies, anthropological measurements, and other genetic markers permitted the Aborigine to be characterized as a distinct racial group differing from either individual or varying combinations of African, Asian, and European groups

(Kirk, 1977). The data supported the concept that the virtual geographic isolation of the ancestors of the contemporary Aborigine over many thousands of years resulted in an identifiable unique population, the Australoids. This theory regarding the isolation of the Australian continent is obviously reinforced by the unique fauna found only in Australia. However, the possession by the Aborigines of some traits by physical anthropology, including tooth size, blood group, and serum protein gene frequencies unique to some of the natives of New Guinea and other islands north of Australia, supports the belief that early ancestors of the Aborigine migrated to the continent from islands further north (Brace, 1980; Curtain, 1972; MacIntosh, 1977).

In their native state, the Australian Aborigines pursued a nomadic subsistence strategy of hunting and gathering, with each of the approximately 500 tribes occupying a generally delineated territory (Elkin, 1964). The scarcity of food, both plant and animal, in most of the desert region forced this nomadic existence upon the Aborigine. This was further accentuated during times of drought which periodically occurred in the interior. The duration of these drought periods is impressive. In his study of Aborigines of the Rawlinson Range area in the summer of 1963, Macfarlane (1978) noted that: "There had been no effective rain for five years." This impoverishment of the land resulted in the need for the bands of Aborigines to travel widely. It has been estimated by Long (1971) that as much as 200 square kilometers were required to support one person, and groups that he encountered in the late 1950's had knowledge of areas exceeding 52,000 square kilometers. In the course of the exploitation of wide geographic areas for food, the men were usually occupied in the pursuit of large game while the women and children gathered edible plants and small animals. However, in their search for food, each individual gathered opportunistically any variety of food encountered (Thompson, 1939). Small quantities generally were eaten raw on the spot, large quantities were brought back to the camp to be shared.

It is important to emphasize that not all Aborigines lived in the impoverished desert climate of the interior. Those natives living along the coast or adjacent to one of the many rivers draining the peripheral areas of the continent had a rich environment which resulted in decreased expenditure of time and effort to acquire sufficient tood. As a consequence, the minimal personal property typical of the Aborigine of the interior was greatly expanded by the natives living in the more fertile regions, as illustrated by a greater variety of weapons, hunting and fishing nets, canoes, baskets, bags, and other items (McCarthy, 1977).

For the unacculturated Aborigines of the interior, it was estimated that vegetable foods contributed over 70 percent of the diet (Meggitt, 1957), but this figure was challenged to be excessively high (Peterson, 1978). Comprehensive lists of food eaten by the Aborigines were reported by Abbie (1960), Campbell (1939), Irvine (1957), McArthur (1960), Macfarlane (1978), Meggett (1957), and Thompson (1939). As summarized by Macfarlane (1978): "Aborigines, in essence, ate anything which was digestible by an omnivore." Earlier, Campbell (1939) commented: "It may seem a sweeping statement to those who have had no opportunity of seeing these aborigines in their natural environment, but it is truth to say that the Australian aboriginal eats as food anything at all that is safely edible. This includes various roots, leaves, nuts, fruits, grass seeds, grubs, ants, beetle larvae, frogs, lizards, snakes, birds, bird eggs, various rodents and all of the marsupials indigenous to Australia." As noted by Peterson (1978), these reports provided insufficient information to permit quantitative contribution of the various foods to the diet. The marked variability of the different species further impeded clarification of the chief staples, whether plant or animal.

Analyses of various plants consumed by the Aborigine have been reported (Peterson, 1978). Some sodium was found in nearly all the seed specimens with the quantity ranging from undetectable to as high as 180 mg per 100 g of the original sample for one type of seed (*Portulaca overacea*). Obviously, the actual quantity of sodium provided by such foods would depend upon the quantities ingested and, as noted (Peterson, 1978), most observers failed to rank the various foods regarding their quantitative importance to the diet. Furthermore, there was a high seasonal irregularity to the availability of the different foods, both plant and animal, comprising the full menu of the Aboriginal. This not especially surprising fact has been described frequently (Irving, 1957; McArthur, 1960; Peterson, 1978; Thompson, 1939).

Another natural source of sodium for the Aborigine was in the various animals which were consumed. The methods of preparation of animal food by the Aborigine were well described by Campbell (1939), Flannagan (1853), McArthur (1960), McCarthy (1960), and Thompson (1939), and resulted in the optimal retention of fluids, minerals, and other substances. Basically, preparation consisted of a preliminary removing of scales, feathers, and fur, the latter often singed off initally in the fire. With the exception of small animals, the viscera were removed, the site of incision closed, and the entire carcass thrown upon the fire. For large animals, such as the kangaroo or wallaby, the body cavity was filled with hot stones and the exterior of the carcass covered with hot sand, ashes, and coals. All observers are consistent in reporting that the cooking time was sufficiently short that the meat would be considered grossly undercooked by acculturated standards. Nevertheless, the technique was satisfactory for the palate of the Aborigine and resulted in the maximum retention of fluid, minerals, and other substances. The habit of the Aborigine to drink the fluid and blood which accumulated within the cooked carcass provided an additional source of minerals.

Finally, it should be emphasized that the Aborgine, in a manner similar to the Yanomamö, frequently cooked both vegetable and animal foods directly in hot ashes. The ashes adhering to the cooked food served as a further source of dietary minerals. Although these would include some sodium, potassium would be the dominant cationic mineral contributed by that source.

In a discussion of the dietary characteristics of the Walbiri tribe of western central Australia, Meggitt (1957) made the following comments:

"Seeds comprise by far the major part of Walbiri vegetable foods. Almost all are collected by women, ground on stones to form a coarse meal which is worked into an unleavened, unsalted paste with the addition of water. In most cases, this is cooked in the ashes to make a heavy, tasteless, evil-looking but nourishing cake. Presumably Walbiri derive sufficient salt for their needs from the uncooked xerophilous plants they eat, for I have never seen them use any native-produced mineral salt, and rarely do they accept the salt offered them on stations and settlements."

Parenthetically, this distaste for salt was subsequently replaced by an avid salt appetite in groups observed at a later date (Macfarlane, 1973, 1978).

In a comprehensive review of food, food values, and food habits of the Aborigines, Campbell (1939 observed: "Sodium chloride is well provided by his wide range of diet and his water supplies." The review also provided analyses of the mineral content of water from samples of springs from the southwest margin of the Great Artesian Basin and of the Flinders Range.

Sodium chloride and sodium carbonate were both present in varying quantities in these samples of potable water.

The hostile desert environment of a major portion of the interior of Australia placed maximum stress upon the Aborigine for maintenance of homeostasis for extracellular fluid with its constituents of sodium chloride and water. Because sources of water were often 30 to 50 miles apart, the Aborigine had to travel long distances in high summer temperatures while progressively acquiring deficits of water (Campbell, 1939). Numerous observers commented on the ability of the Aborigine to drink as much as two liters of water in less than a minute (Campbell, 1939; Macfarlane, 1973, 1978).

Homeostatic regulation of water and electrolytes during summer was systematically studied in the Aborigine by Macfarlane (1973, 1978). Study sites were located in central desert areas of the Australian outback. Subjects consisted of three groups of Aborigines at three levels of acculturation. The most primitive, the Ngatjatjara of the Rawlson Range area, lived with minimal European food supplements brought by truck at three month intervals. The most acculturated, the Pintubi at Warawiya, had liberal access to store-based food supplies of the adjacent government station; they obtained flour, sugar, salt, tea, and dried fruit to complement their indigenous diet. The third group, the Pitjantjatjara of the Kalka area, were considered to be at a midpoint in acculturation between the two previously described groups. Members of the expedition served as controls. General health of the three groups was good and the nutritional state of natives from infancy to adults appeared adequate.

Observations on urinary sodium and potassium excretion were made on overnight specimens collected from males (Table V-1). The data indicate generous concentrations of sodium in subjects of all groups. As anticipated, higher values were found in the samples of the most acculturated subjects. Concentrations, however, remained far below those of the European controls. Unfortunately, there are no reported data reflecting sodium balance in Aborigines subsisting solely on their native diet. The available information suggests that replacement of native foods by those of acculturated sources resulted in progressive increase in sodium intake. Studies of sweat sodium and potassium in representative subjects of the groups showed progressive decreases in potassium/sodium ratios with progressive acculturation. Macfarlane interpreted the data to reflect successive reductions in aldosterone activity with increased salt consumption.

In his summary, Macfarlane concluded:

"The overall picture of these hunter/gatherer hordes, as they made contact with European foods and culture, was that of well fed infants and adults. Traditional foods involved less hunting and gathering as acculturation increased. Flour, sugar, tea, beef and salt replaced the kangaroo and grass-seed food increasingly.

"Streptococcal and staphylococcal infections of nasal sinuses, conjunctivae, and bronchioles became universal. Changes in blood pressure, sweat concentration, sweat suppression and body fat took place as more Europeanisation occurred. The gross obesity of residents near towns did not accumulate in the desert peoples since they retained a hunting and gathering tradition to obtain the interesting components of their dietary."

The accumulated data support the concept that Australian Aborigines in their native habitat ingested sufficient sodium from their natural diet and water sources to permit sodium homeostasis without use of mineral salt or substances of high salinity. The available evidence is compatible with an adaptation for sodium homeostasis to be identical to that observed in contemporary societies and in other primitive groups who have been investigated. The projection of Australian Aborigine population which at the time of first contact numbered approximately 300,000 substantiated the success of this group in adapting to a harsh and demanding desert environment in which an absence of dietary salt was only one facet.

Perusal of the reports on the Aborigines and on the inhabitants of the many island groups of Oceania indicate a wide distribution of cultures living in virtual salt-free environments (Figure V-1).

Table V-1. ADULT MALE ABORIGINES AND CONTROLS: OVERNIGHT URINE CONCENTRATIONS OF SODIUM AND POTASSIUM*

	Na mEq/l ± SE	K mEq/l ± SE	K/Na
1963 European	191.7 ± 5.9	99.8 ± 14.4	0.52
1969 European	140.0 ± 13.4	79.2 ± 5.3	0.56
1963 Ngatjatjara	53.4 ± 3.8	68.5 ± 11.1	1.28
1963 Pitjantjatjara	80.5 ± 5.1	36.1 ± 5.7	0.45
1966 Pitjantjatjara	44.7 ± 5.1	25.5 ± 7.1	0.57
1969 Pintubi	74.1 ± 5.4	20.8 ± 1.4	0.28

*From Macfarlane, WV, 1978, with permission of publisher.

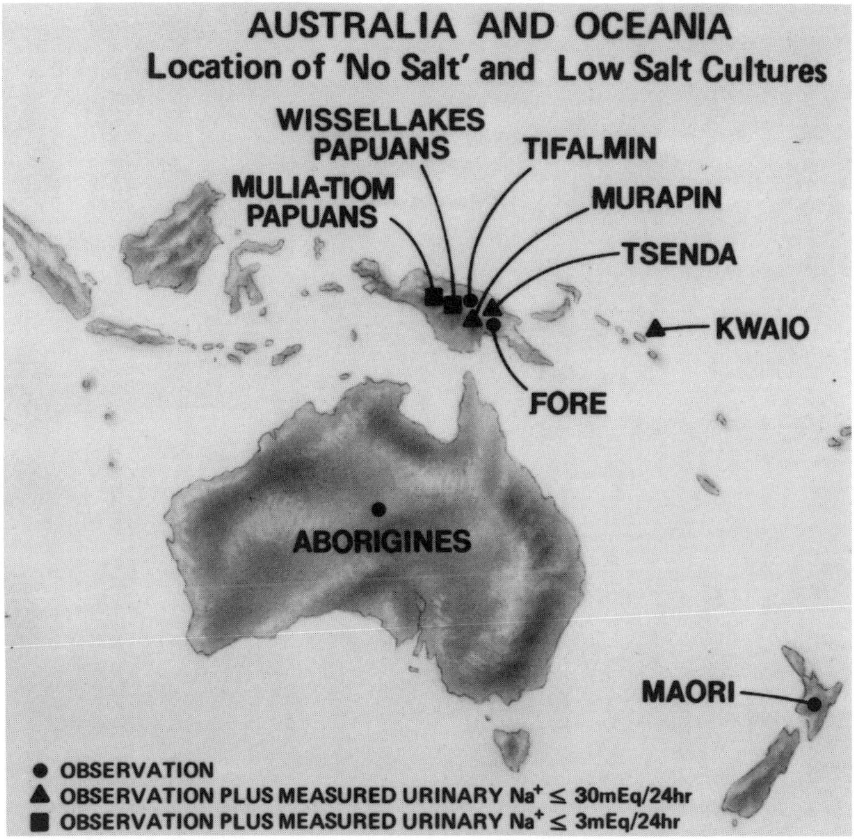

Figure V-1: Location of 'no -salt' and low salt cultures in Australia and Oceania.

VI. Africa

The availability of salt on the continent of Africa varied from extensive salt deposits in regions of the Sahara Desert to essentially non-existant sources in the vast land areas south from the Western Plateau of present day Mali, Niger and Chad. In coastal areas, mining of natural salt deposits and salt-boiling operations provided local supplies of the mineral. In the interior, early European explorers frequently commented on the absence of salt in the native diets in their descriptions of dietary customs. Several warrant review.

In 1791, the Dutchman, Pieter Brand, discovered the Berg Damara tribes living in the Auas Mountains and the headwaters of the Swakop River in the interior of present-day Namibia. These nomadic people were primitive hunters and gatherers of *veldkes* (wild edible vegetables). Hunting was a group activity of the men, and the game was divided on return to the village. A description of the dietary habits of these people was reported by Vedder (1928):

"The Berg Damaras of the veld, i.e., those who are still untouched by European influence and live according to the manner of their fathers, subsist on the wild fruits of the veld and the spoils of the chase.

"When large game is killed, custom prescribes that the hunters, upon their return to the village, drag it past all the huts of the village and then lay it down in the centre of the village at the holy fire, where it is divided - the men who are entitled to a seat at the holy fire receiving special accomodation.

" . . . the flying termites pour from their nests on warm and calm evenings and they are harvested with the aid of fire and carried to the villages in bags. The termites are then dried, pounded and eaten as porridge. It is apparent that they are nourishing food. The stores of a certain ant, which gathers large quantities of grass seed in its subterranean storage chambers as a provision for the rainy season, are also attacked. When rain reaches a portion of such stores, the ants carry the most seeds to the surface in order to dry them in the sun and thereby reveal the location of their stores to the Berg Damara, who digs into the ground at such spots. The stores of the ants are removed by the bucket, roasted and eaten.

"Another article of consumption, frequently obtainable in great quantities, consists of stamped locusts. These locusts travel in large swarms and descend at night. In the cool nights they grow stiff and are easily gathered with the aid of fire. They are also roasted and then sorted. A porridge is prepared by the addition of water and provides a nourishing meal of a sour taste.

"The meal is prepared by roasting large pieces of meat and bulbs, as well as lizards, mice and birds in hot ashes or by boiling them in water, without the addition of salt."

The Bushmen of the Central and Northern Kalahari Desert and the northern half of Namibia were described as subsisting upon a nomadic hunting and gathering existence, roaming in small bands of 50 to 60 individuals over a relatively fixed area of land delineated by natural landmarks from the land of adjacent bands (Dornan, 1925, Fourie, 1928, Shapera, 1930). For these people, the critical geographic features of each hunting territory were the waterholes near which encampments were always made. Movement from the perimeter of one waterhole to another was dictated by exhaustion of edible plants and increasing scarcity of game in the area. Usually several months were spent at one site, with the band then migrating to another waterhole, again remaining until food supplies became difficult to procure. For the Bushman, housing consisted of an open type of shelter constructed of tree branches, twigs, and straw. This served as a windbreak and was abandoned upon decampment. Material possessions were few, consisting of clothing, decorative ornaments, hunting equipment for the men, and items associated with food preparation and eating for the women.

The Bushmen were scattered over an area of approximately 60,000 square miles (Fourie, 1928). At least 50,000 square miles of this area was unknown and uninhabited except for the Bushmen whose numbers were small and estimated to be between 2,500 and 3,500. As in many primitive groups, men were responsible for the hunting and snaring of game, preparation of weapons, and skins for clothing. Occasionally, they assisted the women in fetching wood and water. The women built the huts, collected *veldkos,* made the fire, gathered wood, fetched water, prepared food, and manufactured eggshell beads for ornaments, etc. They were also responsible for keeping the camp clean.

The all-encompassing dietary pattern of the Kalahari Bushmen was vividly described by Dornan (1925):

"The Kalahari Bushmen are practically omnivorous. Nothing comes amiss to them. Hunger compels them to use everything eatable, both animal and vegetable. They catch and devour mammals, herbivorous and carnivorous; birds, snakes, iguanas, fish and insects. Practically every living thing is devoured. All kinds of buck, large and small; zebras, lions, leopards, hyenas, jackals, porcupines, hares, rats, mice, birds of all kinds, including nestlings, snakes, poisonous and non-poisonous; tortoises, iguanas, frogs, barbel, locuts, grasshoppers, flyings ants and wild honey, and often the lice on their persons are eaten. In common with many savage tribes some of them seem to have a preference for these little parasites.

"The Masarwas are not particular as to the state of the food they eat. It may be putrid, but it is all one to them: they devour it and seem to suffer no ill-effects. They crack and swallow the contents of eggs that are just ready to hatch, or that are absolutely rotten, with great relish. They never pass the nest of a bird without appropriating the eggs, no matter what state they may happen to be in."

In an extensive description of the dietary pattern of the Bushmen of the Kalahari Desert, Fourie (1928) noted:

"The source of the food supply varies very considerably in different localities. In some it is derived mainly from the vegetable, in others from the animal, kingdom. The Kalahari and northern parts of the territory are rich in both plant and animal life and the Bushmen inhabiting those parts consequently have a fairly well-balanced dietary.

"Among insects, locusts, ants, scorpions, young bees and honey are greatly relished. Frogs, lizards, snakes, etc., are also eaten. In fact, all living animals are eaten with the exception of the mole and the hyena, the former because its winter larder of *öintjes* forms a valuable and easily obtainable addition to the supplies of the Bushmen and the latter because it eats human corpses.

"After an animal has been shot it is followed by the hunter until it expires or until nightfall when he returns to the *// gãus* (camp). The following morning the whole community takes part in the search for the carcass, as the previous day's tracks had in all probability been effaced during the night by other animals. The searchers spread out on a wide front and keep a very sharp lookout for the presence of vultures. After the carcass has been found it is skinned by the men. The belly is then opened and the entails removed and cleaned. Bags are made from the stomach and into these the blood is collected.

The animal is next cut up and, after this has been done, the liver is roasted and eaten by the men. The skin, if suitable for the purpose, is cut into sandals, bowstrings, etc., on the spot. . . . After having kindled the fire the *gei-khoib* instructs one of the men - the one who has shot the animal is excluded from doing any work - to open the bones and collect the marrow. The blood and the marrow are placed on the fire in separate pots and at the same time some of the meat for the men is also cooked. As soon as the latter is ready for eating the *gei-khoib* removes a piece from the pot and "tastes" (*tsa-tsa*) it. This is done by holding it between the teeth and fingers and cutting off and eating a morsel or two. The meat is now safe for the members of his group to eat. The cooked meat is then pounded with a stone, teased between the fingers and thrown into the pot containing the blood. The melted marrow is next stirred into the mixture of blood and meat. The resulting dish is known as *≠koms*.

"The implements and utensils which are used in the collection and preparation of food are very few in number. Vegetable food is dug up with a sharpened stick, 2 to 5 feet in length. *Öintjes, // ñoun* and other similar plant foods are roasted in hot ashes covered with cinders. Ants (Bushman rice) are dealt with in a similar manner and then recovered again by means of a sieve of grass matting. Locusts are either roasted or boiled. Frogs, etc., are sometimes roasted over the fire on a wooden spit (braaistok) stuck into the ground. Birds, snakes, small antelope, etc., are prepared by placing them in a hollow made in the ashes with a flat paddle-shaped wooden scoop and covering them over with live coals. The meat of larger animals is either cooked or roasted. Among the tame partly disorganised groups any sort of receptacle such as a paraffin tin serves for cooking purposes. The more primitive groups use clay pots bartered from the neighboring Bantu. Roasted plant food is eaten whole or in the form of soup or porridge after being pounded up in a wooden mortar or on a stone and mixed with boiled food.

"Food is eaten direct from the pot or from bowls made of wood or the hide of big game. Many groups nowadays make wooden spoons. Generally, however, either the hands or tortoise-shell spoons are used in eating.

"Every part of an animal is eaten or made use of for some purpose or another. Nothing is allowed to go to waste by those groups which, through possessing dogs, find it comparatively easy to kill game. The camps of the latter are generally littered with bones, etc., whereas among the wild Bushmen even the bones are broken up and eaten. "

The dietary habits of Bushmen of the Namib Desert and of the Central and Northern Kalahari Desert were reported by Shapera (1930):

"The life of the Bushmen is one long struggle for food. For their subsistence they rely entirely on the natural products of their environment: their animal food is obtained mainly by hunting, and occasionally fishing, while their vegetable food consists of edible plants, roots, and fruits growing wild in the veld.

"The Bushmen will eat almost anything that can be eaten. Of animal foods the favourite is game of all kinds, when it can be obtained, and they are also very fond of hare, spring hare, guinea fowl, korhaan, partridge, ostrich, and other birds, as well as birds' eggs. Fish too are eaten wherever they can be caught, and among the Bushmen of the Okavango swamps are a staple article of diet. Anteaters, ant bears, tortoises, porcupines, bull frogs, snakes, and lizards are greatly relished, while among insects locusts, scorpions, beetles, young bees and honey, termites, flying ants and ants' eggs are also eaten. In fact all kinds of living animals are made use of as food, with the almost universal exception of the baboon and the hyena - the former 'on account of its being so like a man,' the latter 'because it eats human corpses.'

" . . . numerous varieties of edible roots, berries, cucumbers, tubers, melons, and ground nuts appear in great profusion during and after the rainy season, when they form the principal part of the daily menu.

"Much of the food is eaten raw, but the Bushmen know how to prepare and cook it. Each family prepares its own food. Cooking is done chiefly by the women, assisted by the children; in exceptional cases the men also may cook. Wild cucumbers, nuts, bulbs, and similar plant foods are baked in hot ashes covered with cinders. A bright fire is made and allowed to die down, a hole is scraped in the ashes with a flat, paddle-shaped wooden scoop, the food put in and covered over. It is then eaten whole or in the form of soup or porridge, after being pounded up in wooden mortars or on a stone and mixed with boiled blood. Birds, snakes, small antelopes, etc., are baked in the same manner; ants are similarly treated, and then sifted through a mat of loosely-woven reeds, while locusts are either baked or broiled. Grewia berries are sometimes eaten as picked, stone and all, sometimes dainty kinds of meats are roasted over the fire on a wooden spit stuck into the ground."

The dietary habits of the Bushmen living in the Southern Kalahari Desert were described by Maingard (1937):

"Bushman is still attached to the life of his forebearers . . . by the fact that they still retain their nomadic habits to this extent whenever posible.

"They do not take meals at fixed times, eating whenever they feel inclined. Usually the big meal of the day is eaten just after sundown. Cooking methods are primitive. I had an opportunity of observing something of their cooking methods when out hunting in the veld. A kill was made and we camped near the kill. The Bushmen straightaway began eating the fresh meat, braising it on the coals of the camp fire. The meat so cooked is half raw, but they have no difficulty in tearing it to pieces with their strong jaws. They can consume astonishingly large quantities of meat in this way. . . . . . .The use of salt appears to be unknown to them."

Limited data on the mineral content of the foods of the Bushmen are available. Although meat, as prepared and eaten by the Bushmen (Fourie, 1928), provided the maximum salt content of the animals, the availability of game from hunting varied in extreme with only minimum quantities obtainable during the wet season when the herbivores could graze over wide areas with little or no limitation to the availability of water. The Bushmen were quite selective in their choice of *veldkos,* only nine species constituting three-quarters of their vegetable diet (Wehmeyer, 1969). Three of these the mangetti fruit (*Ricinodendron rautanenii)*, the tsi bean (*Bauhinia esculenta*), and the sa tuber (*Vigna dinteri)*, were collected in the habitat of Bushmen in the Dobe area in the northwestern region of Botswana, and the mean nutrient and electrolyte composition determined (Wehmeyer, 1969). The sodium content was only slightly more than 2 milligrams per 100 grams of original sample in the nut of the mangetti fruit. Although the seeds of the tsi bean contained an average of 89 milligrams of sodium per 100 grams of raw nut, the uneven geographic distribution of the plant and its seasonal availability reduced its importance in contributing to the daily diet of the Bushman. The sa tuber contained 16 milligrams of sodium per 100 grams but was considered to be a minor food component. Overall, the low content of sodium in these edible plants was not unexpected and parallels findings in most vegetable foods.

A study of blood pressure and salt intake was made of the !Kung Bushmen in the northwestern Ngamiland, Botswana near the Aha Hills (Truswell, 1972). Located in an isolated desert climate, these Bushmen were considered to live close to their native unacculturated state. In typical nomadic fashion, they migrated from water hole to water hole during the dry season of April through October each year. Regarding the habits of this group, it was noted:

"The Bushmen have no alcohol but they smoke tobacco. They have very little salt. There are no deposits of salt in the area and the principal means for obtaining salt is to walk to Tsumkwe, 30 miles away in southwest Africa, where the Administration has established a settlement for the !Kung Bushmen of the South West African side of the border."

Twenty-four hour urine specimens were collected from six Bushmen of this tribe and from two of the expeditionary controls in 1967 and again from four of the Bushmen of this group and from three controls in 1968. Results of the electrolyte analyses are summarized in Table VI-1.

The mean sodium excretion of the controls was similar to those of contemporary populations. In the Bushmen, the mean excretions were 31 mEq per 24 hours in 1967 and 29 mEq per 24 hours in 1968. It appears plausible that in the absence of salt from a trading post, the mean values would be lower than those found.

No information was given about the actual intake of salt by individual Bushmen constituting the study group, but obviously at least two had very low urinary sodium values and the group as a whole displayed findings considered by the authors to be evidence for a low salt diet.

Further north in Equatorial Africa, the interior was characterized by a near total absence of salt. However, appetite for the mineral served as the basis for brisk trade of various items including slaves, gold, ivory, cloth, corn, and cotton. The nature of this exchange was well described by Park (1883) and Schweitzer (1939).

Mungo Park was a Scotsman trained to be a surgeon, but his name is remembered for his explorations of inland West Africa in the regions of the headwaters and midcourse portion of the Niger River (Park, 1883). His unfortunate demise on his second expedition in 1806 at the age of 34 years of a drowning accident at a point on the River Niger in the country of present-day Nigeria thwarted his attempt to complete the last few hundred miles down the river to the Atlantic Ocean (Lupton, 1979). Nevertheless, his detailed descriptions of the topography, the peoples, their subsistence, and the local fauna and flora gained for him an esteemed name among lists of the explorers of the interior of Africa. Park's observations of trade patterns within the various villages along the route of his explorations provided a vivid picture in respect to the absence of sources of salt in the Equatorial rain forest.

In the small village of Pisania, located on the banks of the Gambia River in the present-day country of Gambia, Park provided a detailed description of the goods bartered between European and intermediate traders and the native black population. Manufactured goods including firearms, ammunition, iron wear, cotton caps, glass beads, amber, and other trifles were exchanged for slaves, gold dust, ivory, bees wax, and hives. Slaves, however, constituted the principal commodity. Park wrote:

"In payment of these articles, the maritime states supply the interior countries with salt - a scarce and valuable commodity, as I frequently and painfully experienced in the course of my journey. Considerable quantities of this article, howver, are also supplied to the inland natives by the Moors who obtain it from the salt pits in the great desert, and receive in return corn, cotton cloth and slaves."

Further in the interior at a large village on the Falemë River, Park described methods of catching and preserving fish for sale to inhabitants of the Moorish countries to the north of the Senegal River:

"The small fish were taken in great numbers in hand-nets, which the natives weave of cotton, and use with great dexterity. The fish last mentioned are about the size of sprats and are prepared for sale in different ways; the most common is by pounding them entire as they come from the stream, in a wooden mortar, and exposing them to dry in the sun, in large lumps like sugar loaves. It may be supposed that the smell is not very agreeable; but in the Moorish countries to the north of the Senegal, where fish is scarcely known, this preparation is esteemed as a luxury, and sold to considerable advantage. The manner of using it by the natives is by dissolving a piece of this black loaf in boiling water, and mixing with their *kouskous*."

The absence of sources of salt in the interior was noted by Park in his comments upon the territory of Bondou:

"From the central situation of Bondou, between the Gambia and the Senegal Rivers, it has become a place of great resort, both for the slatees*, who generally pass through it on going from the coast to the interior countries and for occasional traders, who frequently come hither from the inland countries to purchase salt.

"These different branches of commerce are conducted principally by the Mandingoes and the Serawoollies who have settled in the country. These merchants likewise carry on a

---

* native slave traders

considerable trade with Gedumah and other Moorish countries, bartering corn and blue cotton cloths for salt, which they again barter in Dintilla and other districts for iron, shea-butter, and small quantities of gold dust."

Scarcity of salt is further documented by Park in reporting the use of milk by the Foulahs, native inhabitants of the Bondou territory:

"But although milk was plentiful, it is somewhat remark-markable that the Foulahs, and indeed all the inhabitants of this part of Africa, are totally unacquainted with the art of making cheese. A firm attachment to the customs of the ancestors makes them view with an eye of prejudice everything that looks like innovation. The heat of the climate and the great scarcity of salt are held forth as unanswerable objections; and the whole process appears to them too long and troublesome to be attended with any solid advantage.

"Wawra is a small town surrounded with high walls, and inhabited by a mixture of Mandingoes and Foulahs. The inhabitants employ themselves chiefly in cultivating corn, which they exchange with the Moors for salt.

"Early next morning (July 14th), having first returned many thanks to our landlord for his hospitality, while my fellow-travellers offered up their prayers that he might never want, we set forward, and about three o'clock arrived at Moorja, a large town, famous for its trade in salt, which the Moors bring here in great quantities, to exchange for corn and cotton cloth."

In his account of the Mandingo tribe in Kamalia and the surrounding region, Park commented on certain dietary and other customs:

"The beverages of the pagan negroes are beer and mead, of each of which they frequently drink to excess. The Mohammedan convert drinks nothing but water. The natives by all descriptions take snuff and smoke tobacco; their pipes are made of wood, with an earthen bowl of curious workmanship. But in the interior countries the greatest of all luxuries is salt. It would appear strange to a European to see a child suck a piece of rock-salt as if it were sugar. This, however, I have frequently seen, although, in the inland parts, the poorer class of inhabitants are so very rarely indulged with this precious article, that to say *a man eats salt with his victuals* is the same as saying, *he is a rich man*. I have myself suffered great inconveneience from the scarcity of this article. Long use of vegetable food creates so painful a longing for salt, that no words can sufficiently describe it."

Park further described the method of preservation used by these people for fish:

"The fish are taken in wicker baskets, all with small cotton nets, and are preserved by being first dried in the sun, and afterwards rubbed with shea butter, to prevent them from contracting fresh moisture.

"It (gold) is also found in great plenty in Jallonkadoo (particularly about Boori), another hilly, but by no means an unfertile, country. It is remarkable that in the place last mentioned (Boori), which is situated about four days journey to the southwest of Kamalia, the salt market is often supplied at the same time with rock-salt from the Great Desert and sea-salt from the Rio Grande; the price of each, at this distance from its source, being nearly the same. And the dealers in each, whether Moors from the north or negroes from the west, are invited thither by the same motives - that of bartering their salt for gold."

The widespread distribution of salt as a major item for barter appeared in further observations by Park:

"A small quantity of gold is likewise employed by the slatees in defraying the expenses of their journeys to and from the coast, but by far the greater proportion is annually carried away by the Moors in exchange for salt and other merchandise. During my stay at Kamalia, the gold collected by the different traders at that place for salt alone was nearly equal to one hundred and ninety-eight pounds sterling; and as Kamalia is but a small town, and is not much resorted to by the trading Moors, this quantity must have borne a very small proportion to the gold collected at Kancaba, Kankaree, and some other large towns. The value of salt in this part of Africa is very great. One slab, about two and a half feet in length, fourteen inches in breadth, and two inches in thickness, will sometimes sell for about two pounds ten shillings sterling; and from one pound fifteen shillings to two pounds may be considered as the common price. Four of these slabs are considered as a load for an ass, and six for a bullock."

Albert Schweitzer provided additional vivid descriptions of the lack of salt in the African interior in the country of Gabon (1939):

"According to the information of the old people here whom I still knew at the beginning of my activities, there was formally no salt whatsoever in the interior. This changed in 1874 when the whites came to this land and handled the traffic. European salt was shipped in small packets of a few pounds.

"Salt was greatly coveted as a medium of exchange, for none was to be found in the interior. The natives seasoned their food with potash, which they prepared by burning some small, fleshy-leaved marsh plants. Before the coming of the white man, the coast people carried on a very remunerative trade with those of the interior by the medium of sea salt. This was gradually displaced by the salt the white men brought in sacks, so that the coast natives lost their previous profits. In order to retain their salt trade and along with it trade in general, they did all they could to frighten and stop Europeans from penetrating into the interior of the country. Hence it was that, whereas the coast at the mouth of the Ogowe was known since the end of the fifteenth century and had long been visited by white traders, it was not until about 1870 that they first came up the river!

"Salt is still the currency best appreciated in the interior. In remote districts where the nearest trading post is many days' journey distant, the people have no use for money.

"According to du Chailu's account, for a young slave he saw delivered a Portuguese dealer gave a keg of rum containing a hundred liters, a few yards of cotton cloth, and a number of glass beads. The payment for a young woman was a gun, a large copper kettle, sixty yards of cotton cloth, two pieces of iron, two machettes, two mirrors, two files, two plates, two bolts, a small barrel of powder, a few beads, and some tobacco. These were prices at the coast. In the interior slaves might be purchased for much less. There a young man would cost four pounds of salt, a copper kettle, a few yards of cloth, and a few glass beads.

Schweitzer further discussed the indigenous foods available to the native Africans:

"Equatorial Africa, as I have noted in *On the Edge of the Primeval Forest,* possesses no indigenous fruit-trees or fruit-bushes. The banana, the yam, cassava, the sweet potato and the oil-palm are not indigenous, but were introduced from the West Indian Islands by the Portuguese. In those districts of the interior to which these useful plants had not yet penetrated, the natives had for food, in addition to what they obtained by hunting and fishing, only certain roots and the nuts of a few forest trees. When their hunting and fishing were unsuccessful - as often happened - famine ensued. The inhabitants of these famine districts, especially near the sources of the N'Gournie, regarded the country near the coast with its plantations - not to speak of salt - as a desirable paradise for their children.

"From those same famine districts there used to come to my Hospital people who were earth-eaters. As a result of hunger as children they had formed the habit of eating earth and continued it even when they had enough to eat.

"When explorers or business men undertook trips to the interior, numbers of natives offered themselves to paddle their canoes. These made use of the opportunity of buying slaves up country at low prices and bringing them down under the white man's protection without having to pay customs dues to the chiefs through whose territory they traveled.

"In the interior slaves were commonly bartered for salt. The prospect of reaching a country in which there was salt made many of them forget their sadness over the loss of their homes and the parting from their families. Trader Horn reports that once on the River N'Gournie he met some large canoes in which the slaves were looking quite merry because they were hoping to get salt and salt fish at the coast. But very many slaves suffered terribly by being forced to go to a strange land."

An overview in respect to the nearly generalized absence of salt in Equatorial Africa and the southern most portion of the continent has been graphically presented (Bloch, 1963) (Figure VI-1). Native substitutes for the mineral were widely used. For the vast Equatorial zone drained by the Congo River and extending eastward, ashes of burned plants served as condiments. Further east toward the shores of the Red Sea and in the southern tip of the continent below the Kalahari Desert, blood of cattle constituted a standard dietary item. Simultaneously, within eastern areas of Africa both above and below the Equatorial Belt in the region of the 30th degree longitude, this custom was shared with the consumption of cattle urine as sources of sodium salts. Thus, extremely large land areas were devoid of accessible sources of the mineral, but exploitation of local substitutes by the indigenous people obviously was successful in terms of human survival and population expansion.

In summary, the observations and reported data document that distinct tribal groups living in various parts of Africa existed and survived in no-salt cultures prior to acculturated contact. As in other unacculturated groups, a major source of sodium would appear to be meat of the herbivores available by hunting during the dry season but of limited accessibility during that part of the year characterized by numerous rains and wide dispersion of game. Other potential sources probably providing a minimum contribution to the diet included sodium in the vegetable plants and in the cooking ashes adhering to roasted food. For some tribes, ingestion of cattle blood, either alone or in combination with urine from these animals, served to augment sodium intake. In Equatorial Africa the combination of an absence of sources of salt and the unmasked salt appetite of the interior natives resulted in widespread trade of the mineral for various exchanges including slaves, gold, and agricultural products. However, from the descriptions by Park and Schweitzer, it is evident that the mineral was often unavailable in various parts of the interior.

A panoramic perspective in respect to native exploitation of locally available substitutes for sodium salts in the form of plant ashes or cattle blood and urine (Figure VI-1) emphasizes the unavailability of the mineral in large portions of the continent. Yet, this absence of the crystalline compound in the interior was unaccompanied by observed adverse effects upon the health of the individuals. The observations further suggest that these peoples had fully active and adequate physiological means for preservation of salt balance in environments characterized by the extremes from arid deserts to tropical rain forests.

Table VI-1. MEAN VALUES AND RANGES OF 24-HOUR URINARY EXCRETION OF SODIUM AND POTASSIUM IN !KUNG BUSHMEN OF THE DOBE AREA OF BOTSWANA*

Subjects	Year	Sodium (mEq/24 hr) Mean (Range)	Potassium (mEq/24 hr) Mean (Range)
Bushmen			
N=6	1967	31 (8-48)	70 (31-93)
N=4	1968	29 (2-64)	103 (48-168)
Controls			
N=2	1967	212 (179-245)	68 (52-84)
N=3	1968	147 (96-172)	61 (43-75)

*Modified from Truswell (1972) with permission.

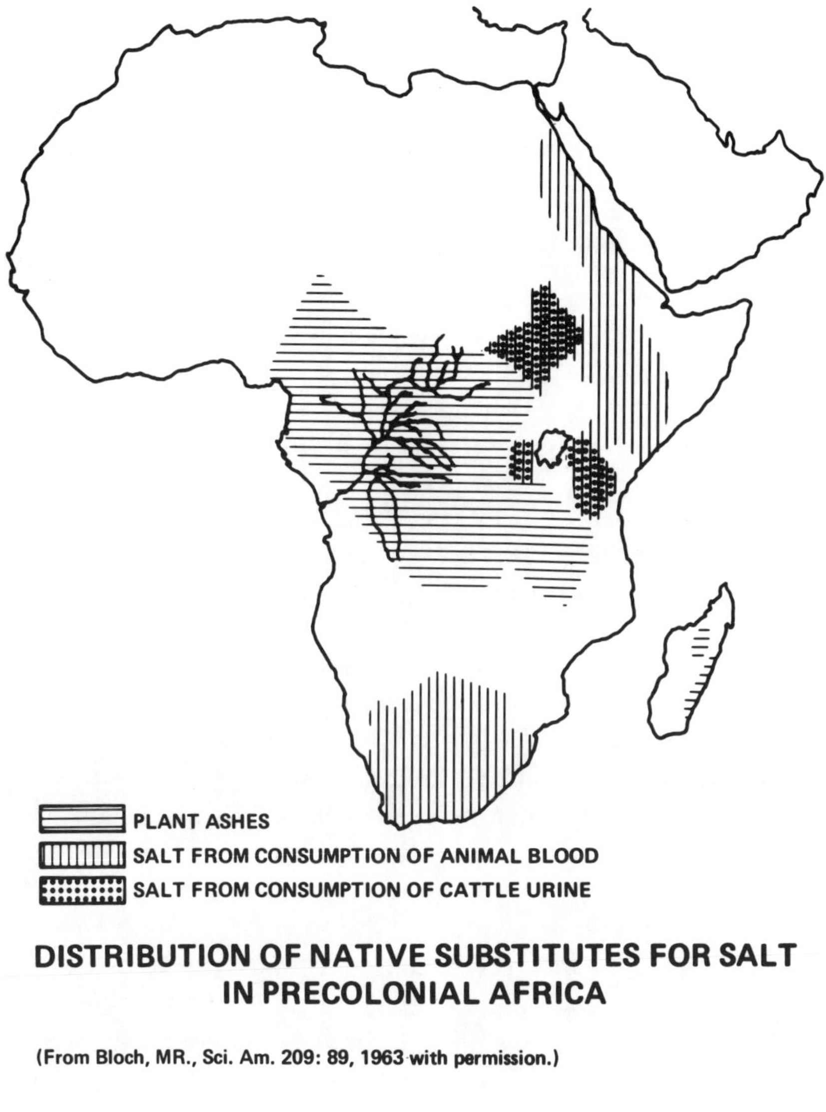

Figure VI-1: Distribution of native substitutes for salt in precolonial Africa. (From Bloch [1963] with permission).

VII. Philippines:

The report in 1971 of a previously unknown primitive group of stone age cavemen living in the Philippine Islands was greeted with great interest by an intrigued audience throughout the world. The Tasaday were accidentally encountered by an itinerant hunter and herb gatherer in the unchartered, mountainous tropical rain forest of the southern Mindanao Island in 1967. The first formal contact with outsiders did not occur until 1971 (MacLeish, 1972; Nance, 1975). This small band numbering only 24 individuals were cave dwellers with one of the most primitive cultures ever described. Their technology was limited to the stone ax, stone scrapers, digging sticks, and bamboo knives. The bow and arrow, sling, and traps for animals were unknown by the Tasaday. Fire was made by use of wooden drills. Neither hunting nor agriculture was practiced by these isolated primitives. Food was gathered daily from the tropical rain forest surrounding their cave dwellings. The wild yam, biking, constituted the staple of their diet. From the numerous streams in their habitat, they collected tadpoles, frogs, and freshwater crabs. These were wrapped in leaves and put adjacent to hot coals for cooking. Additional foods included grubs found within rotted logs, palm fruits, wild bananas, and other edible fruits and leaves unidentified by botanists.

The Tasaday had no source of salt and had never seen the mineral until it was shown to them by members of the early exploring party (MacLeish, 1974; Nance, 1975). Their language had no word for salt, nor for taro or cassava. The good general health and stamina of the Tasaday living in a no-salt culture were points of discussion by those making the early contact with this band. Nance noted:

"The apparent lack of salt in their diet was puzzling. Rebong, the expeditionary physician, said that 'the total absence of salt means that the body tires quickly, becomes prostrate, and eventually dies'. His speculation was that the Tasaday got the necessary amounts of sodium chloride from plants. We knew that they ate many more fruits and plants than we had been shown so far. Elizalde could offer no certain explanation, but he believed that nothing was impossible regarding the Tasaday. 'Who knows exactly how or why they function so well in here? This is a new ball game. You've got to open your minds and treat everything as new. It's the only way you'll get anything more than surface understanding. Maybe they don't need salt.'"

It is parodoxical that despite conscious recognition that the Tasaday displayed no evidence of ill health from an absence of dietary salt, a sack of this mineral constituted one of the gifts to the Tasaday! Man at times rejects what is a fact but inexplicable in terms of prior experience and present understanding.

The time interval of isolation of the Tasaday from other native tribes can represent only a speculation. The existence of cognate words between the language of the Tasaday and that of the adjacent Manubo Blit tribe suggests a possible origin of the parent group for the Tasaday.

No genetic data are available to confirm this premise, but language linkage usually parallels anthropometric and genetic data. The use of the firedrill is all but forgotten by other endogenous tribes while the lack of knowledge of agriculture by the Tasaday suggests the schism to have occurred many centuries in the past. Current estimates place this isolation between 500 and 1,000 years ago. Ultimately, a firmer interval for this time span may be made by various investigative techniques, especially those of a genetic nature.

In summary, the observations thus far completed upon this tiny aggregate of 24 individuals permit a firm characterization that they represent a no-salt culture. Initially, they also represented a group living successfully on a diet distinguished by an absence of meat of avian or mammalian sources.*

---

*The authenticity of the isolation of the Tasaday has been questioned in subsequent reports (noted by Farquhar, M., *Washington Post,* October 27, 1996).

VIII. Salt-users in the Pre-Columbian Era

The use of salt among certain unacculturated groups at the time of initial post-Columbian contact is well documented. There is, however, confusion regarding valid data on the use of salt in the pre-Columbian diet. This confusion is well illustrated in the following discussion of preservation of food by salt among various western Amerindians (Kroeber, 1941):

"It has been generally assumed that the Indians merely dried their meat and fish, without salting it. Probably this point should have been inquired into, rather than being assumed and left out of most of the lists. In two blocks of lists preservation by salting appears, apparently through having been volunteered by informants. For 16 Northeast California lists Voegelin has these entries . - 'Fish salted': +, Trinity Wintu, Valley Maidu; (+), Foothill Maidu, Atsugewi; -, all others. 'Dried meat, salted or plain'": all +, except - for Eastern and Western Achomawi and McCloud Wintu. For the Central Sierra, in 13 lists, Aginsky gives 'Fish' (and again separately 'Meat')" 'stored in baskets with salt'": +, 2 Northern Miwok groups; all others, no entry. It may be that this was a native habit in some areas. The matter should certainly be reinquired into. However, it is more than eighty years since the white man overran the localities in question; and until there are further data which have been cross-checked for the point, I incline to believe that an occasional informant confused post-Caucasian and pre-Caucasion practice. If the habit were old, more of the 150 informants in the salt-using area would presumably have forced it on the recorder's attention."

For North Amerindians east of the Missisippi, there are several descriptions of the production and use of salt. The Taensa Indians of the lower Mississippi Valley lived on a lake created by a prior diversion in the course of the Mississippi River. The village was located in the vicinity of present-day Tensas Parish, Louisiana. This tribe was related to the larger group of Natchez Indians. The first report of the Taensa appeared in the account by Tonti, a member of de la Salle's expedition of 1682 (Swanton, 1911). Tonti's observations were recorded by the then ill de la Salle:

"This lake has the shape of a crescent. The village of the Tinsas is on this lake. M. de la Salle sent thither three Frenchmen with the Akansa. They were well received. The chief of the village sent twenty canoes with provisions, such as corn, dried fruits, and salt. There were also figures of men, bison (*boeufs*), stags, alligators (*cocodrilles*), and turkeys, made of dough, with fruits. When asked if they had saline waters they motioned toward the setting sun and that it was necessary to go in that direction. When asked whether in descending the river one found salt water they replied by turning the head to indicate that they did not know, never having been there. They also indicated that there were evil nations there which would eat the French. Four Loups (Mohegans?) became frightened and remained in this village, and the two Akansa returned home. M. de la Salle did not go to the village at all."

In 1686, on his second expedition to the sea, Tonti again visited the Taensa. A third visit occurred in 1690 as Tonti made the Taensa village his point of departure in an expedition westward in search of de la Salle. He wrote that 12 Taensa started with him, but by the time he arrived at the village of Natchitoches there were 30. He noted:

"The chiefs of the three nations (Natchitoches, Ouasita, and Capiche) assembled and before they began to speak the 30 Taensa who were with me got up and, leaving their arms, went to the temple to show how sincerely they wished to make a solid peace. After having taken their God to witness they asked for friendship. I made them some presents in the name of the Taensa. They (the Taensa) remained some days in the village to bargain for salt, which these nations got from a salt lake in the neighbohood."

Swanton commented: "We know from many other sources that the trade in salt between the Caddoan tribes (which included the Natchitoches Confederacy) and the tribes along the Mississippi was anciently a brisk one."

In his famous expedition of 1682, de la Salle made no contact with villages of the Tunica then located near the Yahoo River in southwestern Mississippi since these Indians were enemies of the Arkansas and Taensa. However, he probably passed near their villages or at least some of their hunting camps in northeastern Louisiana, as Swanton noted:

"One day two Indians joined him (de la Salle) loaded with salt which they said they had obtained at one of these Tunica towns, and it may very well have been that Tunica were encamped there at the time, since du Pratz mentions a place near the Ouachita whither tribes from all parts assembled at certain seasons to make salt. A large part of the salt obtained by the Mississippi tribes, however, appears to have been purchased from Caddoan bands, for French travelers several times encountered Natchitoches bringing salt to the great river for sale."

In his expedition of 1778 to the northern portion of present-day eastern Texas, De Mezieres commented on a "rancheria" of Quitseis Indians living in the general vicinity of the Grand Saline River of Van Zandt County in eastern Texas (Bolton, 1914):

"Going north I found after eighteen leagues' march a rancheria of Quitseis Indians numbering twenty warriors, who, having separated from the main body of their nation, have settled here, attracted by a broad and fertile valley, in which they maintain with profit their cornfields and droves of horses. They have nearby the additional advantage of many salines on which they draw not only for their own use but also to sell. They also constantly kill many deer, using the flesh for food and selling the skins. The road that leads to this delightful place is over steep and rocky hills, deep glens, creeks, lakes and bogs, which, taken with the excessive rains, caused us such difficulty that only the zeal and valor of our Spaniards could overcome it."

For the western portion of North America, data on salt intake are provided by the culture element distribution list in studies of 179 particular groups of Amerindians inhabiting the northwestern and southwestern areas of the United States (Kroeber, 1941). Quite discrete lines could be drawn between the southern portion of the study area where salt was used almost without exception and the northern portion of the study area in which, almost without exception, neither salt nor substances of high salinity (ashes of a particular salt marsh grass) were used. This line, described previously, commenced on the Pacific shore at the mouth of the Columbia River and proceeded south and southeast to turn lastly eastward across the Snake River. The Indians in the southern portion of the study area used salt or, if not available, ashes of a grass with a high salt content.

Further north the Indians living in the vicinity of the Salt River on the north Alaskan coast obtained crystalline salt from a bed of the mineral exposed a few miles upstream from the mouth of the river (Stefansson, 1922). The salt was then brought to the mouth of the Salt River and was used for trading purposes. Stefansson noted that this served as the source of salt for the entire McKenzie district. The description, however, does not permit a determination of the practice to be pre-Columbian or post-Columbian in time.

Salt Users

To the south in pre-Columbian Mexico, it has been speculated that the geographic sources of salt influenced the distribution of agricultural populations (Bloch, 1963). In support of this premise is the high association of salt sources with the greater population density in the southern portion of present-day Mexico. Bloch also identified sites at which sea water was boiled. These extended along the shores of the Gulf of Mexico south to the Isthmus of Panama.

For South America, extremes of salt availability and of its use existed. The interior of South America could be characterized as having a near total lack of salt sources in a manner similar to Africa. The situation was quite different in the lands of present-day Peru and the adjacent coastal regions extending north into the area of present-day Ecuador and south to include portions of northern Chile.

In Peru, the manufacture, trade, and use of salt by the indigenous Amerindian populations have been well documented. In the Royal Decree of 1577 during the reign of Phillip II, an extensive questionnaire was sent to the regional commanders of the various Spanish governed areas in present-day Peru and in portions of southern Ecuador and of northern Chile (Jimenez de la Espada, 1965). Among the extensive list of 194 questions designed to provide data upon the customs of the Amerindians and the resources of the country, one specific question addressed the availability and use of salt: " . . . if there are sources of salt in said village, or close-by, or wherever they obtain salt from, and anything else they may lack in terms of provisions or clothing." A collation of the responses indicated that salt was mined or obtained by the boiling of water from saline springs. The quality of the product varied from highly pure white crystals to a dirt-diluted brown mixture. Those villages without access to salt commonly traded cotton for the item. Certain villages, such as Cuzco, provided salt for many of the nearby villages.

The extent to which the Amerindians of Peru would go to obtain salt was well illustrated by the inhabitants of San Joan de la Frontera (Jimenez de la Espada, 1965):

"There is, five leagues to the west of this city, a large mountain that is comprised of salt, somewhat dirty and reddish salt . . . and from a hold in said mountain, there extends inward for a league a salt water lake, which must be entered from the side of the mountain through a small 'window' (or aperture) through which no more than one or two people can enter. And they enter with a small, reed boat -- one fears the darkness, because there is no more light than the light that enters through the tiny 'window' and the waters are deep. And those who enter with their boats carry a net in their one hand, a net fashioned from a curved stick, and an iron bar in the other, so that as they arrive toward the frontal wall of the mountain, they smack the crystalline salt with the bar (this is the salt that forms there). They retrieve the falling salt with their net and then they leave -- because they don't dare to wait and give the wall more whacks, because the little boat only holds a little salt, because it has to fit through the window, and also because the blows to the wall stir up the water and endanger them thusly (capsizing) -- so then they return to the small window and take out the salt they have retrieved in the net, returning again and again until they have as much as they want. And this is only for crystalline salt, of which they take very little."

From the collected data, it appears that the Amerindians of present-day Peru and adjacent regions both north and south customarily used salt. Villages without sources of crystalline salt or saline springs routinely traded cotton, corn, and other foods for the mineral.

In New Guinea, as described, three quite distinct products have been used as sources of salt or salt substitute (McKee, 1955).

Salt Users

Those natives of the coastal districts either used sea water or evaporated it to obtain a dried product. Trade of the crystallized mineral was only conducted within a few miles of the coast. At other sites, inland natives produced salt from salt springs. For inland groups having no access to products of the sea or of salt springs, wood ashes containing no sodium chloride served as a salt substitute.

A high salt intake by certain native groups of the Solomon Islands was reported by Page (1974). For the Lau tribe who customarily cooked vegetables in seawater, intake of sodium was estimated to range from 150 to 230 mEq per 24 hours. As previously noted, for other groups of islanders, estimated intake was less than 20 mEq per 24 hours.

In a detailed account of natural foods of the Aborigines living on the coastal areas of Arnhem Land and of their techniques of food preparation, the following comments were made in reference to cooking native yams (McArthur, 1960):

"To cook the roots of *Dioscorea sativa* L. var. *rotunda* F. M. Bail., stones 3-4 inches in diameter were heated, and an oven made on the hot sand by placing the yams (which had previously been cooked on an open fire for a few minutes) and the heated stones in alternate layers . . . . On one occasion the yam was cooked in sea-water. An old petrol drum which had been cast up on the beach was used, and the roots were covered with sea-water and boiled for 50 minutes. The subsequent treatment was the same as usual."

The cooking techniques for meat by the natives from Groote Eylandt were also described. To prepare a sea turtle for consumption, it was observed (McArthur, 1960):

"The normal procedure of the Groote Eylandt men in distributing turtle was for the men to keep the front flippers and share the rest with the women and children. The omental and mesentery fat are perhaps the greatest delicacies, but the heart, livers, and intestines are also highly regarded. The distribution of the offal depends on the man in charge, but usually all sections of the camp receive part. On one occasion the turtle was cooked in sea-water. The treatment with hot stones was eliminated, and the gut was cut away during the dissection of the body. Apart from this the above procedure was carried out, and the flesh and internal organs boiled together for 55 minutes. Some of the larger pieces of meat were cut up to fit into the half petrol drum which was used in the cooking."

The manner of presentation of the observations regarding use of seawater by the Aborigines as a vehicle for the cooking of vegetables or animal foods suggests such usage to be an isolated event rather than customary procedure. Whether the selection was on the basis of convenience or on the basis of preference for the salty seawwater can only be a speculation. In view of its use generating such specific comments by the observer, it would appear to support the former interpretation as more likely. This would also coincide with the general observation of the Aborigine living successfully without dietary salt or substances of high salinity.

It is likely that other groups not yet identified avidly sought and used salt in the pre-Columbian era. Nevertheless, the information reviewed substantiates use of salt as a non-unique cultural phenomenon among a number of unacculturated peoples. The widely scattered geographic sites occupied by these groups favor an independent acquisition of an active expression of salt appetite. The continental isolation of these salt-users from one another and the often adjacent location of non-salt users further emphasize the probably independence of this behavior.

Salt Users

IX. Overview:

A pattern emerges when these observations and studies are considered in entirety. Many of the peoples first contacted in the post-Columbian era could be characterized to be no-salt cultures. It is possible that there were even greater numbers of such cultures, but the contamination of the native diet by the rapid introduction of salt as a condiment and as a preservative probably obliterated the true dietary state of these people. The extremely prompt assimilation of salt into the native diet is well documented (Chagnon, 1980; Hawkins, 1848; Helm, 1979; Holmberg, 1950) and supports the possibility that this premise is correct. However, in reference to low-salt groups, it is likely that a number of these described cultures were, in fact, no-salt societies before civilized contact occurred (Macfarlane, 1970, 1980; Prior, 1980). Others from the reported observations, in part or in toto, were salt users: North Amerindians (Kroeber, 1941); South Amerindians (Jimenes de la Espade, 1965); coastal aborigines (McArthur, 1960); Melanesians (McKee, 1955); and Polynesians (Page, 1974). Thus, those cultures contacted in the post-Columbian era must be considered to be heterogeneous in reference to consumption of salt. In any event, the presence of no-salt and low-salt cultures was not an isolated phenomenon but a frequent characteristic of groups first discovered in the post-Columbian era.

The geographic distribution of the no-salt and low-salt cultures may be better appreciated in pictorial display. The accumulated information of all the observations and studies provides a dimension to the worldwide extent of this practice (Figure IX-1). If the logical conjecture is formulated that the peoples of each culture defined to be no-salt or low-salt groups possessed the required physiological adaptation to survive and thrive in a sodium-deficient environment, the possible extent of the geographic distribution of those groups can be graphically depicted (Figure IX-2). This postulation provides a minimum estimate and, again, the likelihood of an even greater extent of this dietary characteristic should not be excluded. In fact, in the case of groups in South America it seems more likely that the available literature or the sources located in this review failed to identify a far wider geographic distribution of salt free cultures than was the actual fact.

The diverse climatic and environmental extremes represented by the geographic sites of these pre-Columbian low-salt cultures include arid deserts, tropical rain forests, northern plains with alternating blizzards and droughts, northern woodlands, and arctic extremes. Clearly, the absence of salt offered no essential hindrance to the survival and expansion of these ethnically different groups in their native habitat.

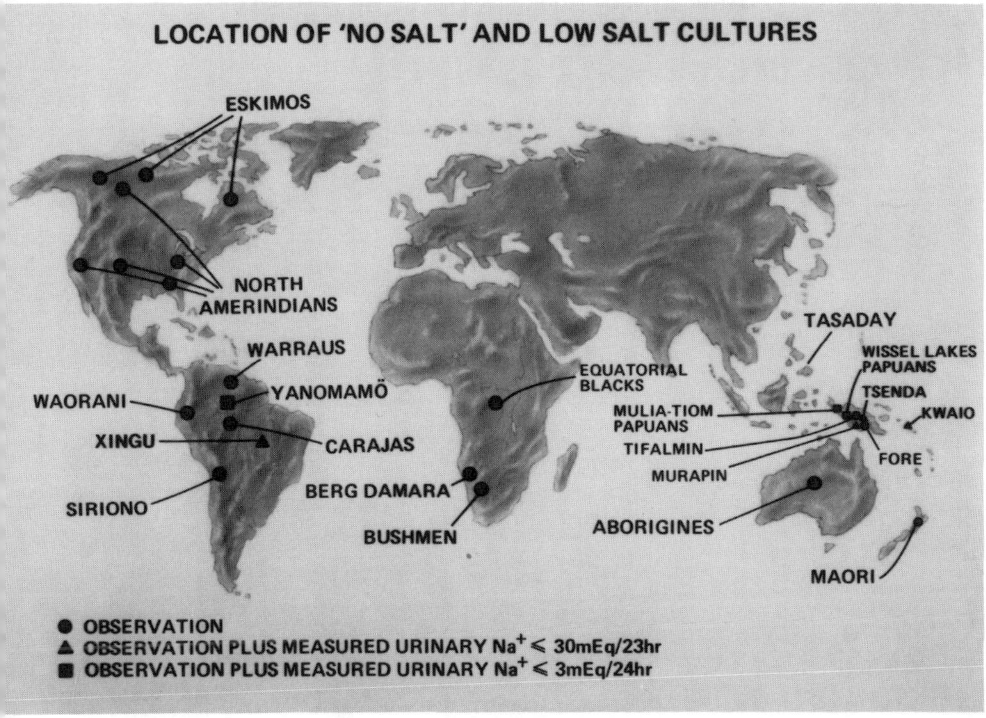

Figure IX-1: World wide location of 'no-salt' and low salt cultures.

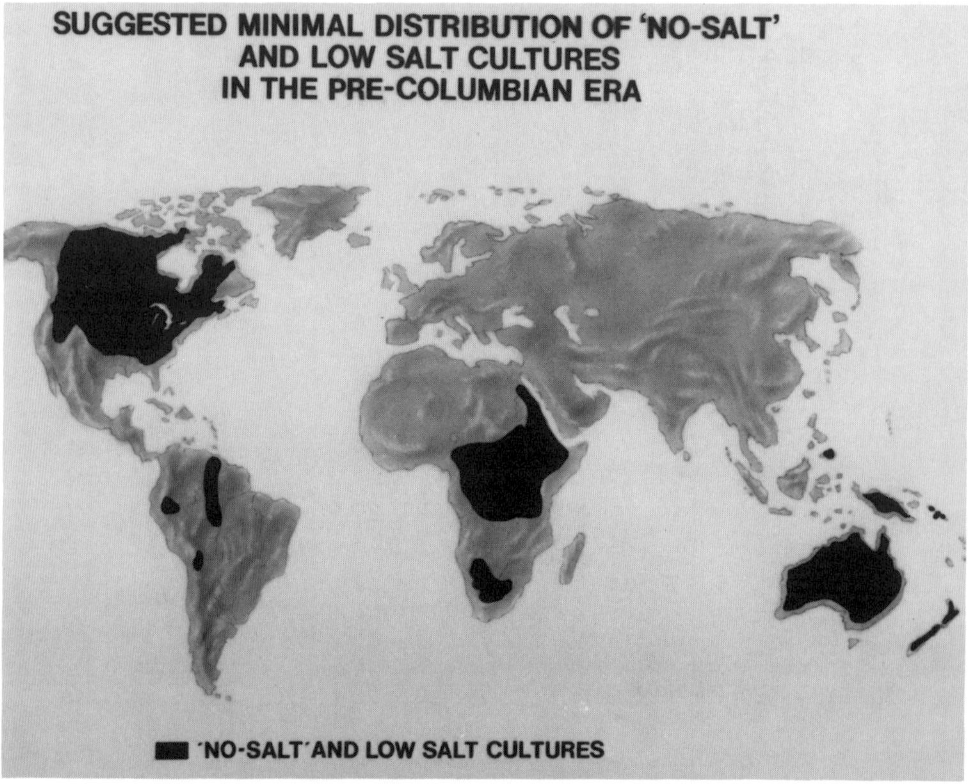

Figure IX-2: Suggested minimal world wide distribution of 'no-salt' and low salt cultures in the Pre-Columbian Era .

X SALT APPETITE IN PERSPECTIVE

The presence of a highly overt appetite for sodium salts is a well-described and documented phenomenon in comparative animals as in man. Any attempt to present a plausible hypothesis for understanding the intricacies of this appetitive behavior must commence with its origin.

In a series of papers Denton and his colleagues described studies of salt appetite in wild and domesticated species (Denton, 1957, 1965, 1969, 1971, 1972, 1973a, 1973b, 1980). These culminated in the authoritative and comprehensive publication, *The Hunger for Salt* (Denton, 1982). This text describes the general deficiency of sodium salts in the soil of many parts of the world, especially the alpine regions and the interiors of the continents. In these areas, sodium is present in only trace amounts in vegetation. Analyses of grasses from the intracontinental Snowy Mountains of Australia, for example, document the paucity of sodium in such samples while similar samples from coastal lands are rich in the element as a consequence of the seawater present in rainfall in these areas.

In the circumstance of a scarcity of sodium ion, phylogenetic emergence of mechanisms to maintain sodium homeostasis conferred an important survival advantage in the successful evolution of vertebrates. In simplest descriptive terms, the optimal adaptation requires a neural component for recognition of sodium need and of environmental sodium sources and an endocrine component for maximum conservation of the ion. The earliest vertebral form in which elements of this system have been found is in primitive bony fishes from which renin can be isolated (Nishimura, 1980). Granulated epithelial cells resembling mammalian juxtaglomerular cells have been identified in primitive bony fishes, teleosts, lung fishes, amphibians, and reptiles. Macula densa cells are first clearly evident in avian species (Nishimura, 1980). The adrenal portion of the axis has been confirmed by the presence of aldosterone in the blood of bony fishes (Denton, 1965; Idler,1959; Philips, 1959).

Evolutionary adaptation of the neural components for sodium homeostasis is documented in the appetitive behavior of various species living in a sodium sparce environment. Alpine kangaroos of Australia confronted by a cafeteria of blocks of filter-paper pulp heavily impregnated with several cationic salts of chloride displayed an unequivocal preference for the blocks containing sodium salts (Abraham, 1973).

Parallel studies were made of the endocrine component of the sodium homeostatic mechanism in a comparison of blood aldosterone and urinary sodium excretion of kangaroos and wombats from alpine and from coastal areas (Scoggins, 1970). For kangaroos living in the alpine regions, urinary concentrations of sodium had a mean of 0.4 mEq with a range of 0.2 to 0.8 mEq per liter. For the wombats of the same area, urinary sodium concentrations were similarly low with a mean of 0.3 mEq and a range of 0.1 to 0.8 mEq per liter. In contrast, samples obtained from these same marsupial species living on the sea coast had much higher urinary concentrations of sodium with means of 268 mEq for the kangaroos and 23 mEq per liter for the wombats. Plasma aldosterone levels were markedly elevated in the kangaroos of the alpine areas. Among the wombats, a slight increase of plasma aldosterone was found in the samples of animals living in same geographic areas, but probably was not statistically significant. As a corollary, the adrenal glands and the areas of the zona glomerulosa, the site of aldosterone secretion, were increased in size in the animals residing in the continental interior.

The data thus indicate that the phylogenetic origin of the neurophysiologic organization of salt appetite and of compensatory mechanisms for sodium conservation originates as far back as the Cretaceous geological period of 70 to 90 million years ago (Abraham, 1975). The integrity and appropriateness of the integrated neural-endocrine system in response to sodium deficits were well documented for higher mammals in the native environments of various wild species and in contrived experiments for numerous domesticated animals (Denton, 1982).

This propensity of wild herbivores to seek out sources of salt is well established in the chronicles of many writers from every continent (Denton, 1982). The known attraction of salt licks and other saline or alkaline sources to the herbivores has been utilized in every continent by man and other carnivores for predatory purposes.

Among the domesticated herbivores, investigation of the adequacy of physiologic mechanisms for maintaining sodium balance when confronted with a dietary deficiency has been best studied in sheep and cattle. In sheep, who are replete with sodium, there was little or no interest in solutions of sodium chloride or of sodium bicarbonate (Blair-West, 1965; Scoggins, 1970). However, when sodium deficiency was experimentally induced by means of a surgically prepared parotid duct fistula, large quantities of both sodium solutions were avidly ingested (Denton, 1957). Simultaneously, the urinary sodium excretion decreased to extremely low values approaching 1 mEq per day with a significant decrease in parotid salivary sodium/potassium ratios. Fecal loss of sodium was found to be less than 2 mEq per 24 hours. These alterations in concentrations of fecal and urinary sodium were associated with increased secretion of aldosterone.

An early study in cattle compared the daily losses of sodium in feces and urine during two levels of dietary intake of the mineral (Renkema, 1962). The low sodium diet approximated an intake of 130 mEq per day (3 g of sodium per day) versus approximately 1800 mEq per day (41.4 g of sodium per day) for the high salt diet. During the lower level of intake, fecal loss of sodium was just under 200 mEq daily, while during the higher level of intake, losses were 752 mEq daily. Simultaneously, urinary concentration of sodium averaged 16 mEq during the low sodium period for two heifers, but only 2 mEq for a milch cow. During the high sodium diet, concentrations of urinary sodium were 148 mEq and 42.6 mEq per liter for the heifers and the milch cow, respectively. Thus, some tendency toward conservation of sodium in feces and urine was evident with this relatively generous sodium intake.

Using a more rigid protocol in the study of hereford steers, approximately 15 months of age, a very low sodium intake of 100 mg per animal daily was contrasted with higher intakes commencing at 3.1 g daily (Morris, 1971). The low diet provided 0.0005 g per kilogram per animal daily. After 166 days on the low sodium diet, fecal sodium decreased to about 3 mEq per day, while urinary losses were at 1 mEq per day. Salivary sodium/potassium ratios were just under 1.5 for the low sodium fed animals, and the ratios were about 23 for those fed 3.1 g or greater of sodium daily. The general health of the steers fed the low sodium diet appeared good, although their weight gain was significantly less than for animals fed the larger quantity of sodium. The investigators interpreted their results to indicate that, in a similar manner to sheep and other animals, the conservation of sodium is effected by increased secretion of aldosterone. This impression was supported by the finding of an increased width of the zona glomerulosa of the adrenal cortex. The authors concluded that the daily sodium requirements for optimal growth of steers is at some point between an inadequate intake of 100 mg daily and that of 3.1 g daily.

Salt Appetite in Perspective

These data on sheep and cattle indicate that both species possess appropriate compensatory measures to adjust for a deficient intake of sodium or for excessive loss of the ion. An important variable was the presence of prolonged lactation which resulted in an obligatory daily loss of significant quantities of sodium. It was reported that 15 g of supplemental sodium chloride were insufficient for lactating cows, but that 30 g of salt daily were ample for the production of at least 20 kg of milk daily (Smith, 1959). The total daily requirements for sodium at such production levels were estimated to be about 21.3 g of sodium per cow daily. Recommendations for dietary requirements place sodium chloride concentrations at 0.46 percent of the dry rations (National Research Council. Subcommittee on Dairy Cattle Nutrition, 1978).

The search for sources of salt or alkali is characteristic of the full spectrum of herbivorous species. A detailed collation of the reports, including both ancient and recent, has been published (Denton, 1982). In brief, the genera included buffalo, cattle, chamois, deer, elephants, elk, marsupials, mountain goats, pigs, rabbits, sheep, and others.

A common theme of the aforementioned data and observations was that the behavior represented an instinctive response to the hunger of salt deficiency. Thus, the actions were considered appropriate and essential to survival of the individual animal and, ultimately, of the species. It is beyond the scope of this discussion to explore the wealth of literature examining the complexities of known, and, as yet unknown, neuroendocrine interrelations and interactions concerned with salt appetite and appetitive behavior directed to avoidance of and correction of sodium deficits. These have been comprehensively reviewed (Denton, 1982).

A second point of considerable importance in developing a hypothesis for a perspective of salt appetite in man is the question of hedonic or need-free salt appetite in animals. Data of interest are available from many species.

Studies of preference for and rejection of sodium chloride solutions were made in nearly 50 individual avian species of several continents. Although the protocols utilized by the numerous investigators were not uniform, in a careful review, it was concluded that "*none* of the species showed any preference for any concentration of saline solution that was tested" (Robizon, 1980). This conclusion also applied to albatrosses who continuously lost salt through their salt excretion glands. Upon induction of sodium deficiency, the birds displayed no discrimination between saline solutions and water (Frings, 1959). Death ensued unless they were given injections of hypertonic saline solution or force-fed salt solutions. Thus, the available data suggest that the sodium content of the natural foods for each avian species in its particular environment, whether high or low in salt, provides sufficient sodium and that an overt appetite for the mineral is not needed.

The common domesticated albino Norway rat displays an interesting preference in relation to distilled water or solutions of various concentrations of sodium chloride (Richter, 1954). These animals, when offered a free choice of distilled water versus solutions of various concentrations of sodium chloride, showed preference for concentrations of 0.8 to 0.9 percent sodium chloride. On the average, these animals ingested approximately 0.5 g of salt per day, which calculated to be 2.0 to 2.5 g per kilogram of body weight. The typically unselected animal (in reference to genetically determined adverse effects of salt in the diet) displayed no insalubrious physiologic effects from this large quantity of voluntarily ingested salt. Furthermore, progressive increments in the quantity of salt added to the diet to comprise up to 35 percent of the weight of the diet was readily accepted by these domesticated rats without a loss of weight. Similar behavior was observed in wild, recently trapped, Norway rats. This high salt intake in both groups of rats was accompanied by parallel increments in distilled water intake. Aversion to increased salt in the diet occurred in diets containing added salt equal to 50 percent and 70 percent, respectively of the weight of the diet. At lower levels, the rats appeared to thrive on quantities approximating 15 to 20 g per kilogram of body weight per day as long as unsalted water was freely available. It appears that the behavioral trait of the domesticated laboratory rat or wild rat in preferentially selecting a high need-free intake of salt is parallel to that of man.

Rabbits represent an introduced species in Australia. In young, wild rabbits captured in the mountains of the interior of Australia, solutions of calcium chloride, magnesium chloride, postassium chloride, and sodium chloride were offered to determine taste preference and need-free intake of sodium chloride (Scoggins, 1970). The diet was considered to contain adequate quantities of sodium chloride. The resultant data were interpreted to indicate that the need-free intake of sodium chloride by the caged wild rabbits was small (0.1 to 0.4 mEq per day per animal) and the data differed quite significantly from those reported on domesticated laboratory and wild rats (Richter, 1954). Of interest was the observation that injections of desoxycorticosterone acetate in the rabbits increased the intake of sodium chloride tenfold, but renal retention of sodium chloride was not observed to occur. Quite a different circumstance was evident when wild, non-captured rabbits inhabiting sodium-poor alpine areas were tested by exposure to wooden posts soaked in various mineral solutions. A clear preference for chewing the posts soaked in sodium chloride and sodium bicarbonate was observed. Similarly, captured rabbits from these sites, when caged before conception, during pregnancy, and, subsequently, for the period of postpartum lactation, demonstrated a preference for sodium salt solutions during pregnancy and lactation, suggesting an appropriate response to these recognized physiologic stresses to sodium blance. (Denton, 1971).

A careful series of studies on the spontaneous intake of sodium chloride in solution by dogs has been reported (Fregly, 1980). Female purebred beagles were fed standard commercial dog food and offered two identical containers with one containing distilled water and the other containing various concentrations of sodium chloride in solution. The dogs demonstrated no spontaneous preference for the salt solutions, with virtually all concentrations of sodium chloride ingested to a lesser extent than water. Additional experiments in which sodium depletion was induced by diuretics also demonstrated no preference for the salt solutions. Substitution of solutions of sodium bicarbonate for the sodium chloride gave similar results. Within the limitations of the small number (five animals) and use of only one breed of dog, the investigators concluded that the dog, unlike the laboratory rat, has no appetite for either sodium chloride or sodium bicarbonate, even when given diuretics. However, balance data for sodium were not obtained. Thus, the evidence must be considered suggestive only.

Using a slightly different protocol, dogs were fed a sodium restricted diet and given furosemide intramuscularly during the first three days of the experiement (Ramsay, 1979). Plasma sodium concentration decreased from 142 ± 1 to 132 ± 2 mEq, and plasma renin activity increased from 3.5 ± 0.6 to 24.5 ± 1.9 mg per milliliter per three hours. When offered water and 0.3 M saline (which is normally rejected by the dog) on the fifth day, preferential selection of the saline solution was observed.

The discrepancy in the results of these two experiments in dogs indicates a need for further studies on this species. The absence of balance data in the first report renders the conclusion of the investigators to be less secure than those of the second authors.

The behavior of herbivores in relation to a hedonic appetite for sodium salts has been extensively and precisely studied by Denton and his colleagues (Denton, 1982). Inasmuch as no parallel studies have been made of other ruminants, the experimental approach and general characteristics of the protocols warrant brief review. The initial series of experiments utilized sheep who were known never to have had access to subterranean saline waters or salt licks. They were fed on a mixed oaten and lucerne chaff diet containing 50 to 100 mmol of sodium per kilogram of dry weight. Free access to water was given. On exposure to a cafeteria of sodium, calcium, and potassium salts in solution for one hour daily prior to creation of a permanent unilateral parotid fistula, the sheep displayed little or no interest in the mineral solutions. The quantity ingested was inconsequential in relation to total mineral intake. Urinary excretion before the surgical procedure was generally above 30 mEq per 24 hours and often approached 90 mEq per 24 hours.

Following the surgical procedure and measured large losses of sodium salts in saliva via the fistula, there was a progressive intake of the solutions containing either sodium chloride or sodium bicarbonate. Urinary sodium excretion fell to very low values and, subsequently, increased parallel to ingestion of the sodium solutions. The authors noted that the specificity for sodium salts was unequivocal, although several animals initially commenced with the potassium chloride solution.

The preciseness of correction of the salivary fistula-induced sodium deficit was measured in two animals over several months. The correlation between the daily salivary and urinary loss of sodium and the voluntary intake of sodium bicarbonate was highly significant ($p < 0.001$).

In additional experiments in other sheep with permanent parotid duct fistulas, the sodium deficit was corrected by instillation of bicarbonate solution through a lumen tube daily. Mean intake of sodium solutions from the cafeteria of solutions was neglible. Upon discontinuing the correction by lumen tube, the voluntary intake of sodium solutions increased to balance losses via the fistula.

It is evident from these experiments that the appetitive behavior represented an appropriate response in these animals to induction of sodium-depleted and sodium-repleted states. Denton discussed an observed variation of hedonic intake of sodium solutions under controlled conditions by individual sheep. However, he further emphasized the reduction in appetite for sodium upon return to the sodium-repleted state following closure of the parotid fistula after several years. Variation occurred among animals, but he noted that in some animals "the cessation of sodium loss results in virtual cessation of sodium drinking, despite hundreds of preceding daily episodes of sodium intake" (Denton, 1982).

The data are consistent with an unpredictable variation of the sheep in their occasional hedonic appetite for salt. The direction of the results in this experimental model more significantly reflects appropriate appetitive behavior to induced sodium-depleted and sodium-repleted states.

It is readily evident that the underlying nature of salt appetite is a more complex phenomenon in the human species when contrasted with non-primate species. A different, and potentially provocative, consideration to this process in modern humans can be approached through phylogenetic reconstruction of primate evolution. The living primate order in which the human animal is assigned consists of six natural groups: (1) the lemurs of Madagascar; (2) the lorises and bushbabies; (3) the tarsiers; (4) the New World monkeys; (5) the Old World monkeys; and (6) apes and humans (Martin, 1992). The interrelationships between these living groups is debated. There is general agreement that they are derived from a common ancestral heritage. On that premise, it is instructive to consider an overview of the evolutionary pathway postulated to lead to modern humans and the other extant primates. In this context, the primitiveness of these archiac ancestors of modern primates is not the focus but, rather, a postulation of the diet required to meet their nutritional needs.

The dietary patterns of archiac forms and subsequent descendants in the primate line can be suggested from the fossil record. Although the data are limited, the remains of bones and teeth permit a reasonably confident interpretation of habitat and diet. The dietary characteristics may be extrapolated to describe the spectrum of nutrients provided. Nutritional requirements of ancient predecessors of extant primates should not differ significantly from those of their modern descendants. Necessary constituents of the diet must provide energy for body processes and physical activity plus the components to build the protein and mineral structures of the body. The five types of nutrients include protein, carbohydrate, lipid, minerals and vitamins. The fossil record suggests that distribution among the first three varied widely. Such diversity is equally mirrored in the dietary selections of primate species of today. Requirements for minerals and vitamins would have had far greater uniformity.

Sodium, as an essential mineral, had to be adequately represented in the diet irrespective of the foods constituting the characteristic fare and their respective quantitative contribution to the total daily intake. By necessity, ancient ancestors of modern humans would have possessed all components of the adaptive physiological processes for efficient recognition and dietary handling of the sodium ion as are present in extant non-primate animals. The environment provided the resources.

In the context of reviewing this evolutionary background, it is generally agreed that primates emerged from archiac terresterial insectovores (shrew-like animals) during the late Cretaceous period between 90 and 65 million years ago (Simons, 1992). The earliest species, *Purgatorius*, living some 65 million years ago, had cheek teeth with sharp cusps compatible with the eating of insects, as seen in extant insectivorous primates, the mouse lemur (*Microcebus*) and the dwarf bushbaby (*Galago demidovii*). By some 60 million years ago, archiac primates had evolved into at least four less primitive genera. Of particular note is the evolutionary trend of teeth towards leaf- and fruit-eating specialization and away from the more primitive dental patterns of their insect-eating predecessors.

The New World primates of today represent a branching of the original simian ancestors some 40 million years ago (Rosenberger, 1992). Throughout their evolution, represented by nearly 40 living species, their lifestyle has been uniquely arboreal. As a consequence, their diets encompass all the opportunities available in tropical rain forests. Descriptively, they can be classified as insectovores, frugivores, folivores, and various combinations. For many, the basic diet often is supplemented by additions of seeds, gums, saps, and flowers. The gastrointestinal tracts of the various species correspondingly parallel the diets. In the mammalian world, the extremes are represented by the true faunivores, with a dominance of the small intestine for absorption of animal protein and by the folivores with expanded stomach and/or caecum/large bowl for bacterial fermentation of the cellulose structure of leaves. The frugivores have gastrointestinal tracts that are intermediate between these two polar positions. Obviously, the various dietary strategies have resulted in nutritional success; otherwise, the species would not survive.

On the other side of the evolutionary ladder, by some 35 million years ago, primates, with dental features similar to modern apes, had evolved from the earlier prosimian forms. These ancient anthropoids, *Aegyptopithecus* and *Propliopithecus,* are considered by some to be the earliest representatives of the *Hominoidea,* the taxonomic unit containing apes and humans. Others disagree and classify them as a primitive catarrhnine form. Of more importance than the classification is the interpretation of the fossilized remains to be those of frugivorous quadrupeds who were adapted to climbing and leaping in the tall canopy of tropical rain forests.

The split of the Old World monkeys, the *Cercopithecoidea,* from the *Hominoidea* (apes and humans) is thought to have occurred early in the Oligocene Epoch (Delson, 1992). The living representatives of the Old World monkey comprise two major families, the *Cercopithecinae* (cheek-pouched monkeys) and the *Colobinae* (leaf monkeys). These vernacular names reflect the major constituents of their respective diets. The former concentrate on fruit; the latter consume leaves as the major dietary constituent. Variations are frequent; some cercopithecine groups eat comparable amounts of fruits and leaves (frugivore-folivores) while seeds constitute a major constituent of the diet of some colobine species. Animal matter, primarily insects and other arthropods, provide 10 to 35 per cent of the diet for various families of the cercopithecines. The capture and eating of small vertebrates is well documented for baboons with prey including very young Thompson's gazelles, young bushbucks, immature African hares plus nesting birds. The observed carnivorous behavior appears to be the result more of a fortuitous event, such as immature animals found hiding in attempted camouflage settings, rather than a deliberate hunting pattern (DeVore, 1963). The activity provides a chance addition of animal meat to the usually vegetarian diet.

In the evolutionary ladder, the extinct simian, *Proconsul*, of the early and middle Miocene Epoch, some 23 to 15 million years ago, is thought to be the last shared relative of apes and humans (Kelley, 1992). This was a monkey-like quadruped with some ape-like features of the hands and the absence of a tail. Fossil remains found in Kenya and Uganda indicate a body size ranging from that of a large monkey to the dimensions of a female gorilla.

The emergence of the ancient ancestors of modern humans is estimated by comparative biochemistry and fossil remains to have resulted from a split from the remainder of the ape family between 8 and 5 million years ago (Wood, 1992). Until recently, the oldest recovered fossils of the earliest form, *Australopithecus afarensis*, fit a time frame of 3 to 2.5 million years ago. New finds dated to between 4.2 and 3.9 million years ago have been interpreted to represent an earlier species of *Australopithecus* (Leakey, 1995). The known geographic locations of these and more modern hominid fossils are currently restricted to eastern and southern sites in Africa. The subsequent more modern hominid, *Homo hablis*, appeared by 2.4 million years ago (Stringer, 1992). It is in about the same time frame that the first recognizable stone tools were manufactured. The distribution of fossils for this period in prehistory extends from eastern Africa to southern sites on the same continent. It is only with the advent of a more advanced ancestor of modern man, *Homo erectus*, that dispersion to Asia and, possibly, southern Europe occurred. Advancement in sophistication of stone tools of flaked forms and larger, multipurpose tools, as hand- axes and cleavers, also became common.

Salt Appetite in Perspective

Approximately 400,000 years ago, the earliest forms of our species, *Homo sapiens,* appear in the fossil record. Representatives of this ancestor of modern man have been found in sites distributed from Africa to the east as far as China and Java to multiple locations throughout present day Europe. Commencing about 200,000 years ago, further evolutionary change resulted in 'Neanderthal Man'. Currently this form is considered to a be a distinct species but not our direct ancestor (Stringer, 1992). Fossil sites for this hominid are quite restricted with locations confined to the continent of present day western Europe. In contrast, fossils of early *Homo sapiens,* in the time span from between 100,000 and 20,000 years ago, are distributed in sites in eastern Asia, eastern and southern Africa, the Arabian peninsula, and multiple locations in Europe.

The diets of these ancestors of modern humans cannot be determined with certainty. The requirements of the dietary background has been succinctly stated: "human beings inherit from their primate ancestors a common set of nutritive needs as well as a set of limited physiological capabilities for intake, absorption, storage and excretion and a sensory apparatus that guides good choice" (Cohen, 1987). In the early phases of hominid evolution, in the interval before development of hunting tools and, certainly, before controlled use of fire, dietary patterns were unlikely to have been greatly different from those of other contemporary primates. The spectrum of foods used by extant primates to satisfy nutritional needs gives a view of feeding strategies potentially available to early hominines. With rare exception, eclecticism prevails. Two species of tree shrews confine their diet exclusively to insects, but the diets of all other living primate species include multiple food options. An inventory of foods consumed by nonhuman primates in their native habitat emphysizes this diversity. In one report (Harding, 1981), food categories are listed as:

A. Animal foods, including vertebrates, crustaceans, and eggs.

B. Invertebrates.

C. Fruits and berries.

D. Seeds and nuts.

E. Soft plant parts, including immature leaves, buds, shoots and flowers.

F. Mature leaves.

G. Roots and grasses.

H. Tree parts, including bark, gum, and decayed wood.

I. Human crops.

Among the food groups, fruit is represented in 90% of all primate diets. It is also the major dietary component of nearly fifty per cent of the surveyed primates (Harding, 1981). Of note is the selection of non-vegetable foods. For all primates, more than one-third of the diet lists include vertebrate or crustacean flesh or eggs. With inclusion of invertebrate species, the per cent of primates deliberately eating nonvegetable foods is above 66%. Quantitatively, these animal foods constitute only small fractions of the total diets of most extant primates.

Of possible greater relevance to the question of the diet of early hominids are the food options selected by the nonhuman members of the *Hominoidea*. The gorilla is almost exclusively vegetarian with mature leaves, soft plant parts, fruits and berries constituting nearly all of the diet. Excurisons into consumption of inverterates occurs, but only to a minor extent. In contrast, the chimpanzee, *Pan troglodytes,* is clearly an omnivorous animal. Although the major components of the daily diet are fruits and berries, none of the other possible options are excluded. The broad categories of food eaten by chimpanzees include leaves and shoots, buds and blossoms, fruits and berries, grains and seeds, husks and pods, nuts, reeds and grasses, vine stems, barks and resins, lichens, galls and larvae, ants and termites, caterpillars and cocoons, birds and eggs, honey, various mammals, minerals, and water. The list of actual floral and faunal species observed to have been eaten by chimpanzees encompass over 200 plant food types and 41 animal food types in one study (Telecki, 1981).

Particular interest has focused on the deliberate predatory activities of these non-human primates. It is well documented that chimpanzees hunt other mammals both collectively and singly. This is not confined to chimpanzees in one location. Reports of field studies of wild chimpanzee troops in Rio Muni, Senegal, Tanzania and Uganda and captive groups reintroduced to a natural setting in Gabon describe hunting behavior for various mammals (Telecki, 1981). Prey species include nine species of primates (baboons and monkeys), four species of ungulates (bushbuck, bush pig, klipspringer and suni), three small mammals (mongoose, giant forest squirrel, and giant rat), plus various birds and their eggs (Telecki, 1981). However, the percentage of total feeding time spent on hunting and eating of fauna is only a small fraction of the feeding time budget. The result of hunting is irregular; some ventures are successful, others are failures. When successful, the kills are observed to be shared among several adults in the community with meat eating periods extending over several hours. Despite the interest in the quantity of meat consumed by chimpanzees and it's contribution to the total diet, firm data are not available. Goodall (1971) observed that a group of 40 individuals captured over 20 different prey animals during one year. It has been tentatively suggested that mammalian meat constitutes either one percent (Telecki, 1973) or from one to three percent of total annual diet (Busse, 1977). A third report gives an estimation of 27 grams per chimpanzee per day (Wrangham, 1975).

Of more importance than the actual quantity of mammalian meat consumed by chimpanzees is the fact that the closest living evolutionary relative of modern man can quite fully exploit the native environment including the deliberate and successful hunting of other mammalian species in a repetitive pattern. The observations document that hunting prowness does not require that an evolutionary difference exist to distinguish early hominids from their postulated nearest living primate relatives. Obviously, the evolutionary ascent brought important changes. A major unanswerable consideration is whether the changes resulted in an heightened or lessened ability to fully utilize the foraging opportunities used by other primates.

It is pertinent also to observe that hunting behavior is not universal in this species. For chimpanzee groups in whom hunting is rarely observed or seldom noted to be successful, no nutritional disadvantages are reported to be accrued nor are reproductive rates lessened (Ghiglieri, 1984). The observations can be interpretated to indicate that vertebrate consumption is not a nutritional essential but possibly a notable behavior documenting a higher level of exploitation of available food sources.

Interest in the ingestion of unusual substances by primates has resulted in detailed observations in several reports. Geophagy, the practice of eating earthy substances, is well described in studies of both chimpanzees and gorillas (Hladik, 1974; Hladik, 1977; Lawick-Goodall, 1968; Schaller, 1963; Wrangham, 1977). The behavior is sporadic and inconsistent. Much variation occurs among different troops of both animals. For the chimpanzee, most of the soil was from earth molded by termites and other insects. Other materials eaten included rotten wood and ashes. On chemical analysis, total mineral content was considered to be insufficient to contribute significantly to nutrition (Hladik, 1974). Specifically for sodium, values ranged from 4 to 104 parts per million of dry sample weight. For the gorillas, soil was eaten at several sites. Samples ranged in sodium content from 160 to 10,980 per million of dry sample weight (Schaller, 1963). It was noted that the ingestion of soil occurred only occasionally by the gorillas and sites rich in minerals often were ignored during passage of the animals near the areas. Again, the inconsistency of the geophagy and the marked variability of sodium content suggest an inconsequential addition to the diet.

A hedonic appetite for sodium salts is a rare phenomenon among primates. An isolated exception may be cited. There is a series of longitudinal observations on a single troop of monkeys (*Macaca fuscata*) living on the Japanese island of Koshima who have developed the practice of washing sweet potatoes in sea water before each bite (Kawai, 1965; Kawamura, 1954). This repetitive behavior clearly suggests a need-free pattern of salt ingestion. Beyond this unique behavior, the observations are convincing that for non-human primates, the sodium ion is present in sufficient quantities in the natural diet, albeit in trace amounts, that all needs are met, even with the increased needs of pregnancy and lactation.

More formalized observations pertaining to salt appetite have been made in another of the non-human primates. In baboons raised in captivity, experimental exposure to varying concentrations of sodium in the diet did not induce a need-free salt appetite (Barnwell, 1986). Instead, irrespective of prior experience with high salt diets, the baboons preferred the diet with the least content of salt. In a second study of captive baboons, no innate hedonic appetite for sodium solutions was found during control observations (Denton, 1993). Following experimentally induced sodium deficiency, a 'robust' appetite for sodium solutions developed with intake of sodium by the baboons resulting in a close approximation to correction of the deficit. Subsequent to repletion, sodium intake fell to control levels without a residual hedonic appetite. These studies affirm that for this species a need-free salt appetite appears to be absent and is not induced under the described experimental protocols.

There are several lessons in nutrition to be learned from appraisal of extant nonhuman primates. The natural and customary diets of these closest relatives of the human animal can be described to be highly diverse in one sense and consistently uniform in another. The overview of the primate diet is that the opportunistic foraging encompasses the complete cafeteria of all possible edibles. Although dominent foods can be identified for each of the various species, the varieties of food items consumed by any one species is widely diverse with inclusions from throughout the native flora and fauna. The uniformity of these diets is in the ubiquitousness of accepted and sought after edibles from both first and second trophic levels. The ultimate consequence of these dietary selections is that all essential nutritional components are incorporated in the chosen natural foodstuffs. The innate instincts for selection of various foods embodies successful response to various needs of the organism, including that for the sodium ion. Ingestion of animal foods is not a constant requirement.

At the time of the split of our earliest ancestor, *Australopithecus afarensis,* from the remainder of the primate family, begining some four million years ago, this precursor of modern humans would have possessed all of the required "physiological tools" to successfully meet the nutritional challenge of the savannas of Plio-Pleistocene Africa. Physical characteristics of smaller canine teeth and of bone structure compatible with bipedalism need not suggest any major dietary differences from those of the contemporary primates of the same time period. The division between plant versus animal foods in the diet of early hominids can only be a speculation. The wear patterns of fossil teeth of these hominids are similar to those of modern nonhuman primates that feed predominently on fruit and leaves. The role of scavenging carnivore discards for meat remains enigmatic. In the absence of controlled fire, digestion of complex macromolecules (dextrins, starches and cellulose) would have been limited and the intake of plants containing various toxic substances (digestability-reducing substances and true biologically active toxins) would have been potentially deleterious (Stahl, 1984). Instead, the focus logically would have centered on foods high in soluble carbohydrates. Fleshy fruits and some underground storage roots (bulbs) would have fulfilled this need. Protein requirements potentially could have been met from a variable combination of plant and animal sources. In reference to hunting, these protohumans were likely neither to have been at an advantage nor a disadvantage in respect to other primates in the successful capture of invertebrates and small vertebrates. It has been suggested that they were simply a step in the evolutionary continuum which began with the hunting and eating of small, mobile insects and and progressed to the predation on small vertebrates (Harding, 1981). They simply exploited the environment for a diverse selection of flora and fauna.

The first appearance of a more advanced hominid, *Homo hablis* ('handy man'), is found in the fossil record dated to some 2.5 million years ago. It is within this time frame that the first crude stone tools appear. There is no current evidence to indicate whether the intellectual ability to make stone tools was also associated with altered behavior resulting in more frequent capture or scavenging of more or larger animals for food. The success of this species is attested to the presisting presence for nearly one million years.

A more sophisticated species, *Homo erectus,* appeared on the evolutionary scene about 1.8 million years ago in East Africa. The stone tools found in association with these hominids in some sites include those describe as choppers and scrapers. These could have materially assisted in the processing of meat and plants. Again, as for earlier forms, no inference can be made in respect to improvement of hunting techniques nor of distribution between species and size of animals gained by hunting or scavenging.

A major advance in exploitation of potential food resources by early humans resulted from control of fire. The timing of this event is calculated from the earliest hearths found in Zhoukoudian, China to date to about 500,000 years ago (Black, 1933). Recent evidence suggestive for use of fire at dates exceeding 1 million years ago has been presented (Sillen, 1990). Fire permitted the processing of complex carbohydrates to more digestible forms and of reducing plants containing various toxic compounds to edible nutrients. At what point in prehistory did cooking meat become customary is speculative. It is not essential for nutritive purposes. The custom of preparing meat with fire before eating by extant hunter-gathers is far from consistent. For many groups, as detailed in earlier chapters, raw meat is considered a delicacy and much preferred. Efforts in cooking, especially of large animals, often is incomplete and frequently inconsistent. The final product, ranging from raw to burned, is seemingly accepted without complaint or rejection. Drying of meat by sun or fire is widely used among these diverse and formerly isolated ethnic groups. The time of origin of this process for preservation of food is unknown.

There are two other diminsions to the advantages of fire for early humans. One is the deterrent value against various predators. The second is the ability to transport fire with its associated warmth which potentially could have assisted in migratory spread of early humans to and through areas with cold ambient tempertures. Remains of ancient hearths and of charred animal bones have been found at isolated sites in Europe as well as in Asia (Black, 1933). More recent hearth sites, dated to about 40,000 years ago, have a much wider distribution. These accompany other evidence of modern humans in multiple locations in western Asia and Europe.

The relationship of the control of fire to evolutionary change of hominids is not firm. For the australopithecines, the relatively large post-canine teeth with deep enamel and thick skull bones for attachment of muscles of mastication suggest the ability to feed on tough, hard plant foods and possibly for extraction of marrow and of the contents of thick kernel nuts. The advent of controlled fire and more sophistocated methods of processing food stuffs would have lessened any disadvantage for the genus, *Homo,* in respect to the evolutionary reduction in molar size and enamel thickness and associated cranial features compatible with smaller bulk of muscles for mastication.

The era of archaic *Homo sapiens* commenced about 800,000 years ago. Whether control of fire aided the dispersion and establishment of this species of our ancestors in distant sites in Africa and the Euroasian continents is strictly conjecture. After a presence of perhaps some 600,000 or more years as indicated by the fossil record, this form becomes extinct as modern *Homo sapiens* becomes the dominent species of the last 100,000 years.

The evolutionary pathway from australopithecus ultimately leading to our modern species is no longer universally accepted to be a straight forward linear ascent in clean genetic steps. Reexamination and reconsideration of the current available fossil remains of our ancestors, their assigned time frame of existance and geographic locations have led to an alterative pathway of hominid evolution (Gore, 1997). The predominent theory has emphysized a linear series of advancing steps from the most primitive to current day Homo sapiens. A remarkably contrary view has been espoused as a setting in which multiple hominid species of our ancestors coexisted in time wih various species disappearing while more sophisticated forms survived. The correctness of this more recent interpretation of fossil data is less relevant to the present consideration than the ultimate attainment of progressively more complex species over time.

A pictorial display considered to represent locations for archaic *Homo sapiens* caught at 125,000 years ago in time identifies more than one-half a dozen sites in present day China, one in India to multiple spots in the southern tip of Africa, extending northward to the northeastern rim of that continent, to multiple sites in western Europe (Gore, 1997). The remarkable presence of fossil remains at such widely dispersed geographic sites over multiple continents requires that the physiological 'knapsack' to be able to adapt to a variety of climatic conditions and of potentially exploitable food sources.

It is evident that 'modern' *Homo sapiens*, accompanied by ever increasingly sophistocated tools and control of fire, progressively migrated to many parts of most continents before the origin of agriculture. There is no evidence that reliance on distinct sources of mineral salts or salt-rich foodstuffs was a requirement for this successful migration. Nor are there compelling reasons or comparative research data to suggest that any evolutionary difference from other primates in the physiological handling of the sodium ion need accompany this migratory pattern. Both archiac and recent ancestors, as well as extant non-human primates, appear to fulfill sodium needs from natural foodstuffs. Meat is not a requirement. In fact, it is equally logical to argue the opposite view - that the various hazards of migration placed an even greater stress on bodily strategies to enhance intake and conservation of the sodium ion.

The preceding discussion would appear to adequately substantiate the premise that archiac and recent ancestors, as well as extant primate relatives, of modern *Homo sapiens* fulfilled needs for the sodium ion with natural foodstuffs. The related proposition: whether present day humans can meet nutritional needs for sodium by natural selection of uninriched foods in respect to sodium salts has been debated for over one hundred years.

In a broad discussion of problems in nutrition, Drummond (1934) aptly provided a dimension to consideration of salt appetite:

"I am inclined myself to think that we must go much deeper than an examination of man's present environment and that we can find the root of the trouble in the complex adaptation which has marked the path of his civilization."

He further elaborated with a quote from Roberts (1897):

"The generalized food customs of mankind are not to be viewed as random practices adopted to please the palate or gratify an idle or vicious appetite. The customs must be regarded as the outcome of profound instincts which correspond to certain wants of the human economy. They are the fruit of a colossal experience accumulated by countless millions of men through successive generations."

Then disagreeing with Roberts, Drummond further commented:

"If this view were correct it would imply that man has retained the natural instinct in the choice of foods which is shown by most wild animals. There is, I submit, abundant evidence that he has not and that civilization has weakened this defense, as it has blunted the acuteness of his sense of smell and hearing. Animals and, to a less striking extent, primitive peoples present many interesting examples of this protective instinct. . . . Sometimes in man we can detect definite traces of the survival of a protective instinct, but even in primitive races it is seldom strongly marked except for certain minerals."

The testing of this premise of the existence of a natural instinct for correct choice of foods by contemporary humans is no less difficult in the world of today than in that of several decades ago. Ready access to salt is a major problem. For nearly all peoples of the earth, the nearly ubiquitous availability of salt (plus the persuasive presence of salt-prepared, salt-preserved, and salt-seasoned foods comprising the usual diets of industrialized societies) confuses and frustrates efforts to investigate the presence of an instinctive salt appetite fulfilling physiologic needs, but avoiding need-free gratification. Some data potentially pertinent to this point are available. The observed instinctive behavior and the learned behavior of two groups displaying independent dietary selection are instructive. These two groups are: (1) members of contemporary societies placed in a circumstance to use instinctive behavior for food selection and (2) members of primitive societies who follow cultural dietary customs of many millennia in duration and who survive, thrive, and propagate without knowledge of the individual biochemical and mineral consiituents of their daily primitive diet. Behavior can be examined for those seemingly without nutritional deficits and for those with apparent deficits. Observations on the former constitute first consideration.

In a classic experiment, newly weaned, breast-fed infants were permitted to choose their own foods in the quantity which they desired from a broad range of commonly used natural foods; these foods were unmixed, unseasoned, and unaltered except a few were given preliminary cooking without seasoning (Davis, 1928). The initial report of this fascinating study involved three white male infants, two of whom were studied for six consecutive months and the third for 12 consecutive months. Of pertinence is that the protocol employed only natural food materials; no canned foods, sugars, or dairy products such as cream, butter, or cheese were offered. These infants entered the study at the ages of seven and one-half, eight, and nine months. Food in small dishes and liquids in small glasses were offered at each meal with the infant actively choosing and manually obtaining the food or indicating his preference to the passively attending nurse. Salt was not used in the preparation of any of the foods, but was offered in a small dish on the tray with all other items. As noted by the author:

> "Salt they ate only occasionally, often spluttering, choking or even crying bitterly after getting it into their mouth, but never trying to spit it out and frequently going back for more, with repetition of the same spluttering, etc."

This activity may be a variant of the antecedent behavior resulting in the overt expression of a salt preference by children of two or more years of age (Weiffenbach, 1980). Of note is the observation by the investigator, Davis, that intake of salt was not a *consistent* choice, but rather an *occasional* selection.

For these infants, their nutritional status on completion of the studies was within the normal range. Their caloric intake approximated those recommended in commonly used guidelines for appropriate age groups of that era. Although the investigator was cautious in interpretation of her data, it was appropriately concluded that the immediate results following six or 12 months of self-selection of diet resulted in adequate, possibly optimal, attainment in terms of height, weight, bone development, musculature, general vigor, developmental milestones, and appearance of health and well-being (Figure X-1).

In a summary of an extension of the same investigative protocol to a total of 15 infants at the ages of six to 11 months, similar data were obtained (Davis, 1939). The author noted that the protocol with choices confined to natural, unprocessed, and unpurified foods reproduced to a large extent the conditions under which primitive peoples in many parts of the world were shown to have scientifically sound diets and excellent nutrition. The author concluded that a permissive environment in which appetite could function without restraint resulted in a successful fulfillment of caloric needs and of nutritional requirements (Davis, 1939).

The limited number of infants in these two studies does not detract from important implications. These infants were breast-fed solely up to the time of entrance into the study and represented a naive and virginal population regarding established habits, prior taste experience, or theories of optimal foods and their appropriate preparation. The observations emphasized the innate survival potential for the human infant presented with a seemingly appropriate cafeteria of natural or minimally altered varieties of food.

Observations of primitive populations provide some insight into the adequacy of their innate dietary selection. For this approach, data on four groups representative of no-salt cultures located at sites remote from one another are reviewed. These groups are the Aborigines of Australia, the Yanomamö Amerindians of South America, the Bushmen of the Kalahari Desert of Africa and the Fore Highlanders of New Zealand. The diets of unacculturated groups include a wide spectrum of animal and plant foods. Such diets have a single unifying characteristic: they are omnivorous for nearly every form of food that is edible. For the Aborigine, it has been stated: "..the Australian aboriginal eats as food anything at all that is safely edible" (Campbell, 1939a) and "Aborigines, in essence, ate anything which was digestible by an omnivore" (Macfarlane, 1978). Schapera (1930) observed: "The Bushmen will eat almost anything that can be eaten." Observation documents similar dietary patterns for other unacculturated groups. Obviously, the food substances available differ among these primitive peoples as a consequence of the varied climatic conditions and the endigenous fauna and flora. Nevertheless, the classes of animal and plant comestibles have a recuring similarity. The spectrum of edible food comprising the diets of these four groups is presented in Table X-1.

On perusal of the varieties of food constituting the native diet of these four groups, it is evident that all utilize nearly every possible type of animal from insects through mammals and a variety of fruits and vegetables, cultivated and wild. With the rare exceptions of certain tribal taboos such as the refusal of the Bushmen to eat the baboon because "on account of it's being so like a man" and the hyena because that animal "eats human corpses" (Schapera, 1930), it can be stated quite convincingly that all animals that move are potentially edible. The usual revulsion of acculturated individuals for insects, snakes, rodents, monkeys and other animals does not exist in these societies. In fact, many of the larvae of several species are considered unusual delicacies by most groups and one species is cultivated in crude fashion by the Yanomamö Amerindians (Chagnon, 1968).

A noteworthy feature of food preparation for consumption by unacculturated peoples is its simplicity. Many plants, some larvae, eggs , and selected parts of animals were eaten raw. Roasting was the commonly used technique for cooking. For small animals (larvae, birds, snakes, rodents and small monkeys), the undressed carcasses were thrown over or covered with hot coals (Fourie, 1928; Campbell, 1939b; Chagnon, 1968; McArthur, 1960; Oliver, 1976; Reid, 1969). With these techniques, the skin of the carcass served as a cooking receptable, and little or no nutrients or minerals were lost in the process. For the Aborigines, the retained juices within the body cavity were considered a delicacy and drunk by them with great relish (Campbell, 1939b). Larger animals were butchered and pieces roasted, but the cooking time in many instances resulted in grossly under-cooked and a semi-raw condition by usual acculturated standards. Such an appraisal would not blunt the appetite of these peoples. Quite frequently, the "steam oven" so well known throughout Oceania was used by the Fore Highlanders for cooking both meat and vegetables for a feast, often held weekly in small hamlets (Sorenson, 1969). The estimates of cooking time were frequently in error, and the pit yielded semi-raw pork and vegetables or an overcooked pile of meat and vegetables. Rare use of the technique was noted for the Aborigine (Campbell, 1939b). The technique also preserved major quantities of nutrients and minerals. Thus, the culinary habits of these representative, no-salt cultures afforded maximum yields of essential nutrients and minerals.

The list of varieties of fauna and flora constituting the spectrum of foods considered edible by these groups closely parallels the list compiled for humans' closest relative, the chimpanzee. There are no significant differences. It is only in the tools used for capture and in fire used for processing selected foods does a difference exist. It is significant to note that despite the verbally expressed desirability for animal protein in the diet by members of these groups, it does not constitute the major component of the diet and frequently is not eaten daily (Chagnon, 1979; Good, 1987).

Of more significance than the smorgasbord constituting the native diet of these primitive groups is the level of nutritional success attained. Assessment of nutritional status commonly employs a multifaceted approach. Components generally consist of knowledge of community consumption of various staple foods, individual diet histories, chemical analyses of major food types, physical examination, and selected biochemical studies. These studies included hemoglobin, hematocrit, serum iron and iron-binding capacity, total serum protein, serum albumin, and levels of various vitamins in blood and urine. Two additional dimensions are the magnitude of physical stamina displayed in the course of everyday living by the people under consideration and their level of reproductive success. These latter two in a highly practical manner document the accuracy of assessments suggested by the other parameters employed in the evaluation of nutrition. For the four groups under consideration, the assessment profiles did not provide all the data customarily gathered in studies of contemporary populations. Nevertheless, the information obtained was useful in evaluating the overall nutrition of representatives of each culture.

One component of the study of nutrition in Aborigines indigenous to Arnhem Land of the Northern Territory of Australia was the collection of data on quantitative food consumption (McArthur, 1960). Four groups were surveyed. Three represented coastal inhabitants and one an isolated inland band. Animal and vegetable foods gathered by all inhabitants of each site were weighed during several days with no correction for food eaten away from camp. Calculations in terms of recommended daily allowances (National Research Council of America, 1948) were made for each of the four sites for total calories and content of protein, calcium, iron, and ascorbic acid. Although there was some variation among the four groups, protein intake per person exceeded 150 percent of recommended allowances per person at all four sites, and estimated caloric intake ranged from 74 percent to 116 percent of the recommended daily allowance. Ascorbid acid was low only in the inland camp, and estimates of calcium and iron intake were adequate in the subjects of three of the four sites. The author concluded that "with only a few exceptions, the diets seen at the four camps in Arnhem Land were well balanced, and they provided amounts of most nutrients comparable with the recommended dietary allowances."

Analyses of the composition of a group of Australian desert vegetable foods were compiled and provided data on caloric value, protein, fat, carbohydrate, mineral, and ascorbid acid content (Peterson, 1978). On perusal of the list, these vegetable foods were low in fat, but high in protein and calories. As would be anticipated, potassium content was high and sodium content low in all samples with the exception of an appreciable quantity of sodium in several seeds. In the absence of data on the volume of intake of specific foods, such as various seeds and roots, the actual caloric and mineral contribution to the diet is unknown.

The physical health and nutritional status of the same four groups of Arnhem Land natives described previously were evaluated by measurements of height and weight and physical examination for clinical evidence of disease or of nutritional disorders (Billington, 1960). Commencing with subjects three years of age, 526 individuals constituting 72 percent of the total population were examined. Comparisons were made with white Australian children for whom data were available. Although the four groups had differing degrees of contact with civilization, the overall findings among them were quite similar. In a comparison of height for age, the Arnhem Land children were slightly shorter than the Australian children. In contrast, although parallel in ascent, the Aborigine children through the age of 15 years had a lower mean weight for height than similarly aged Australian children. Leanness was a characteristic of all subjects of all ages. Obesity was absent. The report noted a general picture of good muscular development and tone in the adults at all four sites. The general build was described to be athletic with well-developed and strong muscles of the shoulders, thighs, and vertebral column. Carriage, posture, and gait were excellent. The Aborigine infants were plump and apparently grew rapidly. Most were walking and had closure of the anterior fontanel by one year of age.

Physical examination of these subjects was considered specifically from the perspective of findings indicative of deficiency of individual nutrients. Inspection of the weight for height curves for the Aborigines versus data for Caucasian Australian females was interpreted to be possibly compatible with an insufficient caloric intake by the female as contrasted to the male Aborigines. The investigators speculated that this could result from a discrimination in distribution of food supplies. The general good health of the infants and children, however, suggested an adequacy of breast milk during the two to three years of breast-feeding. An absence of muscular wasting on physical examination or of other findings suggestive of gross inadequacy of protein intake led to the clinical impression of sufficient protein intake by adult females. The possibility of specific vitamin deficiency (vitamin A, B complex, ascorbic acid, and vitamin D) constituted a component of the physical examination survey of all subjects. With the exception of one elderly woman who was crippled by hemiplegia and showed clinical findings indicative of nicotinic acid deficiency, no clinical evidence for vitamin deficiency was found in the 526 Aborigines.

A less extensive evaluation of the health and nutrition of Aborigines was subsequently reported in a series of slightly over 100 Aborigines inhabiting the region of the Great Sandy Desert in Central Western Australia (Elphinstone, 1971). Males were described as slimly built and sinewy in physique. Two young females of 12 and 15 years were believed to have scurvy on the basis of swollen and friable gingivae, although no other lesions suggestive of scurvy were noted. Similar or other findings suggestive of scurvy were not found in any of the remaining subjects.

A study focusing on hematologic findings of the Central Australian Aborigine included samples of 145 Aborigines inhabiting the Western Desert west of Alice Springs (Casley-

Smith, 1958). The mean hemoglobin level in male Aborigines 16 to 80 years old was 16.4 g and for females of similar ages it was 16.2 g per deciliter. Comparative data on European males gave a mean value of 15.9 g and for females 14.1 g per deciliter. Data on mean erythrocyte counts, mean corpuscular hemoglobin, and erythrocyte diameters were normal for male and female Aborigines from whom samples were obtained.

In another study of natives of the Arnhem Land region, total serum protein values of 7.44 ± 0.54 (S.D.) for 451 Aborigines were slightly higher than those of 7.23 ± 0.42 (S.D.) for 11 European members of the expedition (Hodges, 1960). Since no fractionation of globulins were performed, no data were obtained for the serum albumin level which is a more reliable reflection of total nutrition.

The plasma ascorbic acid levels of the Aborigines of Arnhem Land varied considerably among subjects at the four study sites (Hodges, 1960). In the subjects at two of the sites, the ascorbic acid levels were within the normal range of 0.4 mg per deciliter, and there was no clinical evidence of scurvy. However, 70 percent of the total study population was interpreted to be at a deficiency level. The observation that the mean plasma levels of ascorbic acid of acculturated volunteers receiving only 11 mg daily over many months were 0.03 mg per deciliter (Report of Medical Research Council, 1948) suggests that even though the sources of vitamin C remained an enigma, the mean daily quantities consumed by the Aborigines were sufficient.

Serum vitamin B_{12} levels were assayed in samples obtained from 40 subjects of the Great Sandy Desert (Hetzel, 1978). All 40 had levels well above the accepted normal range for white subjects.

The Yanomamö Amerindians have been the subjects of a series of multidisciplinary biomedical studies which extended over two decades (Neel, 1972; Oliver, 1981). The burn-and-slash agriculture and hunting characteristics were described in Chapter III. Physical examinations were performed in over 600 Indians of both sexes and all ages (Neel, 1976). No stigmata suggesting nutritional deficiencies were found. As noted earlier (Chapter III), the men were of muscular build (Figure III-13) and tolerated long treks over highly irregular jungle terrain with obviously much stamina in an environment characterized by high temperatures and equally high humidity. The general health of mothers and babies similarly was impressively good (Figure III-14). It was only in a few women with advancing age that evident loss of body fat and a general appearance of debilitation were found. The reproductive success of these people has been discussed earlier (Chapter III).

Assessment of the health and the nutritional status of the !Kung Bushmen was the focus of a multidisciplinary biomedical expedition in the Okavango River territory of South West Africa (Bronte-Stewart, 1960). Subjects for study were nomads and were considered by the investigators to represent a late Stone Age culture without knowledge of agriculture or of domestication of animals. Bushmen were assembled at four different sites in the vicinity of their usual range of territory at differing distances from the river. A group of 885 subjects of all ages were inspected and superficially examined for general health and nutritional status, and a smaller group constituting up to 10 percent of the subjects at each site were randomly selected for more extensive clinical examination and laboratory testing. The !Kung Bushmen were described as short in stature with a mean height of 62 $^1/_2$ inches and slender in build with a mean weight of 101 pounds. The women were slightly smaller. The overall assessment was that the state of nutrition was generally good despite the high prevalence of tropical disease as evidenced by splenomegaly in over 51 percent of the subjects. Physical appearance of undernutrition was rarely found in infants or children. Obviously, the nomadic life-style in a desert climate supported the interpretation of a generally robust people.

Laboratory data obtained from a subset of the subjects included mean hemoglobin levels of 14.4 g for males and 13.8 g per deciliter for females. Total serum protein values in 54 subjects averaged 8.31 g with a mean serum albumin of 3.45 g per deciliter. This contrasted to mean values for Capetown Europeans of 6.92 g per deciliter for total serum protein and 3.80 g per deciliter for serum albumin determination. The higher total serum protein values for the Bushmen reflected significantly greater levels of gamma globulin. The investigators concluded that the general health and nutrition of the subjects examined were surprisingly good in the face of chronic parasitosis. However, it was noted that inasmuch as the subjects represented those who had traveled. in some cases long distances, it was possible that elderly and infirm subjects had not made the trek. In any event, available data suggested that the learned dietary patterns of these people in their native habitat did not reflect overt deficiencies of food, minerals, or vitamins.

The Fore Highlanders of Eastern New Guinea have been the subjects of a series of biomedical investigations. Nutrition observations have been the foci of several field studies. An assessment of the traditional native diet was made in the Moke village (Reid, 1969). A daily dietary survey was conducted over a seven day period in three households considered to be typical for the hamlet. Each individual included in the survey was questioned regarding opportunistic food eaten during the daily trek to the gardens. On return from the gardens, the collected food was sorted and weighed by food type (e.g., sweet potatoes, yams, pitpit, greens). For a more detailed individual quantitative analysis, the investigator stayed with the members of one household for an entire day and weighed all the prepared food eaten by each individual. The collected data were analyzed using standard tables of nutritive values both of foods from the New Guinea and Papua Food Composition Tables (Hodges, 1950) and of dried beans from other published data (Platt, 1950). The results were compared with recommended daily allowances for native populations of these areas reported by the New Guinea Nutrition Survey Expedition 1947 (Langley, 1950). The authors concluded that mean daily totals of calories and selected nutrients (calcium, thiamine, and ascorbid acid) were adequate as compared to other New Guinea groups and to the recommended daily allowances. Estimated intake of protein was lower than recommended, but the authors observed that the results represented the overall minimum consumption of protein, since by chance no pigs, which were usually plentiful and generally eaten for several meals weekly, were cooked during the period of the survey. The authors further concluded that nutrition could not be the cause of the kuru occurring in these people.

A review of nutrition among tribes of coastal and inland Western New Guinea has been reported (Oomen, 1961). The daily food intakes tabulated by Oomen were characterized as inadequate to adequate caloric intake based on recommended daily allowance (Langley, 1950); the intakes were highly dependent on the geographic locale with the larger mean values found in coastal groups and in those living close to inland lakes. With rare exception, protein intake was below recommended allowances. Protein intake was relatively more deficient in those with special requirements (i.e., pregnant and lactating women and children with their needs associated with growth). The adequacy of breast-feeding as reflected by infant growth varied from comparing favorably with nutritionally advantaged groups to significant decrements in rate of weight increase commencing after the third month of life. Despite the perceived quantitative and qualitative deficiencies of many of the Papuan communities, little evidence of nutritional pathology was observed. Ooman further noted that long-term population figures for some groups displayed increases with suceeding generations. It would appear that these peoples, although not as affluent in food sources as the three previously considered primitives, were not a consistently nutritionally deprived population.

It is evident that nutritional success was a nearly consistent phenomenon for these four primitive groups following tribal dietary customs of probably ancient origin. The data support Roberts' premise of over a century ago (1897) that dietary patterns respond to instinctive needs of the "human economy".

At the other end of the spectrum from those healthy individuals instinctively selecting foods with sufficient content of salt for nutritional needs are the recognized but isolated instances of appetitive behavior in man to correct for salt deficiency associated with congenital or acquired disease states. One example is that of a three and one-half year old boy with salt-wasting adrenogenital syndrome (Wilkins, 1940). The young boy was admitted to the hospital for evaluation of marked sexual precocity. In the hospital, his appetite was poor, he often vomited, and he died unexpectedly on the seventh day following admission. Subsequent history indicated an overt craving for salt since approximately 12 months of age. In addition to a diet of highly salted foods, the youngster ate from three-quarters to one teaspoon of crystalline table salt daily! An appropriate analogy was noted by the authors between the extreme salt appetite of this child and similar appetitive behavior of adrenalectomized rats to compensate for urinary salt wasting.

Another instance of this phenomenon was a 34-year-old man who had severe Addison disease and who excessively and impressively salted all his foods (Richter, 1943). As described, this man "put approximately one-eighth inch layer of salt on his steak, used nearly one-half a glass of salt for his tomato juice, used salt on oranges and grapefruit, and even made lemonade with salt."

An instinctive craving for salt by individuals with Addison's disease has been observed, but not consistently. Among 64 patients with the disease, 10 (16 percent) had the symptom of salt craving (Thorn, 1942). In later reports (Henkin, 1962; Henkin, 1963), the symptom was present in only 15 to 20 percent of patients with Addison's disease.

The inconsistency of salt craving by man in the presence of salt deficiency may represent individual variation of genetic origin. It has been noted that self-selection of diets is not universally successful in industrialized man (Pangborn, 1944). However, the restrictions imposed by cultural exclusion from the diet of the rich variety of edibles constituting the daily menu of unacculturated primitives constitute a potential basis for this deficiency.

Perverted appetites among animals have long been recognized. These phenomena include coprophagy, infantophagia, placenta eating, and bone eating. In the spontaneous prospective studies in laboratory animals, the majority of these can be ultimately deciphered to represent an instinctive dietary response to a specific nutritional deficiency (Richter, 1943). Similar perverted appetites are described for members of human societies. The literature upon the subject of pica was comprehensively reviewed by Denton (1982).

In man, an instinctive desire for flavoring or seasoning of foods with condiments appears to be universal. Among acculturated societies, prominent additives are common table salt, pepper, mustard, and vinegar. Among primitives a similar spectrum appears. The Fore people of New Guinea used various herbs and barks as condiments (Sorenson, 1969). The Warraus Amerindians of South America routinely used *Capsicum*, a pepper, to season their food (Schomburgk, 1922). Similarly, peppers constituted the major condiment of the Amerindians of the Uaupes River region of the Amazon basin (Wallace, 1853). The Yanomamö Amerindians, on occasion, made a mineral solution from plant ashes which "resembled salt in a vague way insofar as taste goes" (Chagnon, 1980). The widespread use of plant ashes in Africa has been previously noted (Bloch, 1963). In New Guinea, the laborious efforts associated with the production of crystalline minerals from plant ashes (principally potassium salts) and from saline springs have been reviewed earlier (McKee, 1955; Sorenson, 1969). Throughout many of these reports is the underlying theme of satisfying a craving for a salty taste to food. It is particularly important to recall that this appetite is present in groups without evident sodium deficiency.

The development of this desire and of a preference for a salty taste has been investigated in infants of contemporary societies. Neonates are quite indifferent to various concentrations of sodium salts in solution (Weiffenbach, 1980). Infants aged four and seven months did not consume more strained food when salt was added than when the food was unsalted (Fomon, 1970). Data for children above two years of age have been interpreted to indicate both a preference for salted foods and a lack of such preference (Gonzalez, 1983). Possibly the most pertinent finding from the studies was the practical observation that the preference of the parents for salt had a considerable influence on the preferences of the children. An early lack of preference for salt (Fomon, 1970) may not correctly resolve the question.

In studies of subjects of various ages, it has been shown that the ability to recognize a salty taste is blunted with increasing age (Chauncey, 1980). Thus, the older individual requires a greater concentration of salt in a food to achieve a "salty" flavor.

A further factor in perception of saltiness is the salivary concentration of sodium chloride (Chauncey, 1980). Although the concentration of salivary sodium chloride varies with intake, the changes in concentration do not approach the extreme upper or lower variations achieved by the kidney in response to a very high or a very low sodium diet. Nevertheless, if the levels of sodium chloride in saliva are at a high concentration as a consequence of concurrent generous dietary consumption of salt-containing foods, recognition of "saltiness" requires a greater concentration of salt in the food or liquid being tasted. To the limit, then, of customarily achieved high levels of salivary sodium chloride, the individual desiring to gain a salty taste will need a greater concentration of salt in food in order to exceed the higher salt threshold occasioned by the salivary salt concentration.

The overall impression is that several factors in man, including age and concurrent dietary intake of salt, influence the intensity of salt appetite required to achieve satiation. The net effect of these is toward a higher, need-free salt intake.

It is obvious that there is a need for a daily dietary intake of sodium. Dahl (1968), however, lucidly emphasized the distinct difference that exists between *salt requirement* and *salt appetite*. Throughout the long evolutionary process of lower animals and the ancestors of man, a salt appetite and an associated sodium conservation process were essential for survival. The time in history at which man actively sought out sources of mineral salt or substances of high salinity to satisfy a need-free salt appetite obviously can be only a speculation. The absence of a common root word for salt in Sanskrit and its daughter languages has been interpreted to indicate that tribes of migrating Indo-Europeans did not know its use (Schleiden,

1875). Older cultures such as Babylonian, Egyptian, and Chinese, however, knew the use of salt (Kaunitz, 1956). Recorded history from numerous sources and the ages of salt mines and of trade routes for the mineral document the widespread commerce in salt during the later portion of the last several millennia (Benton, 1973). It has been suggested that, among acculturated populations, the practice of using salt in the daily diet commenced in association with the advent of agriculture and a farinaceous diet (von Bunge, 1901). The premise, if correct, would date the need-free consumption of salt back 10 to 12 thousand years before present. Such an interval would span a nearly infinitesimally minute and recent phase of the time interval postulated for the evolution of man (Leakey, 1977). The corollary of that scenario is that the existence of a salt appetite, albeit perhaps not a consciously recognized behavioral action, remained an essential trait for survival until very recent times. That appetite is so firmly fixed in our inherited traits it must be accepted as an immutable genetic characteristic.

A distinction between fulfillment of an appropriate need-associated salt appetite and a need-free salt intake can be gained by observations made of several previously isolated societies. The awakening of a latent hedonic appetite for salt has been described for several primitive groups of diverse geographic and climatic sites. These include the Aborigines of Australia (Macfarlane, 1978), Creek Amerindians (Hawkins, 1848), the Dogrib Amerindians (Helm, 1979), the Sirionо Amerindians (Holmberg, 1950), and the Yanomamö Amerindians (Chagnon, 1980). The rapid assimilation of salt and salted foods into the diet of other primitives throughout the world attests to the inherent nature of a need-free salt appetite in man.

A possible analogy to the hedonic appetite for salt in man is that of drug dependency in the same species. Salt appetite does not in fact differ significantly from drug dependence. One definition of drug dependence which stresses features common to all types of drug addiction provides a provocative consideration (Eddy, 1970):

"As already noted, individuals may become dependent upon a wide variety of chemical substances that produce central nervous system effects ranging from stimulation to depression. All of these drugs have one effect in common: they are capable of creating, in certain individuals, a particular state of mind that is termed *psychic-dependence*. In this situation, there is a feeling of satisfaction and a psychic drive that requires periodic or continuous administration of the drug to produce pleasure or avoid discomfort. Indeed, this mental state is the most powerful of all the factors involved in chronic intoxication with psychotropic drugs, and with certain types of drugs it may be the only factor involved, even in the most intense craving and perpetuation of compulsive abuse. . . . Physical dependence is a powerful factor in reinforcing the influence of psychic dependence upon continuing drug use or relapse to drug use after attempted withdrawal."

It may be argued that such a definition is excessive in reference to need-free appetite for salt. Yet, without a period of adaptation to a very low salt in take, there is a *physical* dependence upon a generous intake of salt. Of pertinence is the fact that physiological adaptation to a minimum sodium intake in the healthy individual requires a minimum interval of 3 to 5 days (Oliver, 1964). In the absence of proved adverse effects of salt intake above physiological requirements, rejection of the analogy is appropriate. However, for over a century the role of salt (sodium chloride) in diseases of contemporary industrialized societies has been controversial. An early espousal of an association of salt intake and disease was the publication entitled "A Treatise on Salt, showing its hurtful effects on the body and mind, on man and on animals, especially CONSUMPTION, as taught by the ancient Egyptian priests and wise men, in accordance with the author's experience" (Howard, 1850).

Over three decades later (1883), Lehmann independently reached the conclusion that the adding of salt to natural foods was unnecessary for man. A diametrically opposite view was expressed by a fellow countryman one year later (Manley, 1884). He stated:

"Salt is the most widely accepted of the condiments. So universal has been its use, that it may be called the 'cosmopolitan' condiment, and so great is the craving for it and relish of it, that we are led to consider the love of it as one of the most potent of our natural instincts, and salt itself as necessary to the health and even life of man. The fact that in no part of the world is salt unknown and unused goes far to substantiate this position. But notwithstanding the general consensus of scientific opinion as to the great value of salt, confirmed as it seems by physiological facts, and it may be added by our natural instinct as well, are found persons who take an oppositive view; and even an authority like Dr. Hassall has made bold to publish the following statement: 'The function' he says 'of chloride of sodium or common salt, is ill understood. It has been asserted that it is necessary for the assimilation of the food, but this seems not to be the case. Salt, in fact, is considered for some to be quite a superfluous addition to most of our articles of food, and nothing more than a condiment. It does not enter into the composition of any of the tissues, but is thrown out of the system in the excretions; and it has been repeatedly shown that some tribes of natives of Africa do not know the use of salt at all, or consider it a luxury and delicacy.' But others have gone further and mentioned that the use of salt is absolutely injurious."

Manley quoted Dr. Howard of some 40 years previously (1850) and stated:

"Unfortunately such extremists will ever be found, and the present age seems particularly prolific of them."

The stimulus for an intake of sodium chloride exceeding physiological need continued to be the subject of much speculation. Several hypotheses have been promulgated and have generated much debate extending over a number of decades. Von Bunge (1901) proposed that extra dietary salt was needed by populations consuming a predominantly vegetable diet. The excess salt presumably was necessary for more effective excretion of potassium. This assumption, which continues to be cited in current textbooks of nutrition, was thoughtfully challenged by Kaunitz (1956). In a provocative discussion well supported by direct field observations of unacculturated peoples concerning dietary habits, Kaunitz emphasized that from the data available for review, it was reasonable to conclude that "this use or non-use of salt by various tribes is irrespective of the amount of agricultural products they consume." This contention was supported by our data on the Yanomamö Amerindians who could excrete in excess of 300 mEq of potassium in their urine daily with simultaneous mean excretion rates of 1 mEq for sodium (Oliver, 1972). In rejecting von Bunge's theory, Kaunitz proposed, but without providing any substantive supporting data, that "salt-eating in some unexplained manner may have facilitated learning." In an expansion of this hypothesis, he proposed that "the quickened pace of a more complicated society demands persons with a heightened responsiveness. Salt may be one of the ingredients producing this effect." Other possible plausible explanations of the hedonic appetite for salt require additional consideration.

The role of salt in the pathogenesis of disease in industrialized societies continues to be widely and spiritedly debated today. This is particularly true for essential hypertension . Two recent publications underscore this dichotomy. Both involve large numbers of subjects.

Data on 52 population groups were initially published by the Intersalt Cooperative Research Group in 1988 and were interpreted to show a highly significant positive correlation between 24 hour urinary sodium excretion and systolic blood pressure. The more recent report (Elliott, 1996) re-assessed the original data for the individual 10,079 subjects with corrections for regression dilution bias. The revisited estimates were interpreted to give even stronger correlation of sodium intake with systolic blood pressure. The data were suggested to provide further support for mass reduction in salt intake for the prevention and control of adverse blood pressure levels in the general population.

On the other side of the ledger, the effect of reduced dietary sodium on blood pressure in hypertensive and normotensive individuals was investigated by a comprehensive, computerized literature-search of studies on human subjects (Midgley, 1996). Reports were limited to trials that had randomized allocation to control and dietary sodium intervention groups and were monitored by timed urinary sodium excretion. Fifty-six studies met the inclusion criteria. The authors interpreted the reviewed data to show a slight mean drop in systolic blood pressure but an insignificant decrement for diastolic presssure in the hypertensive individuals. For the normotensive subjects, a mean decrease of 1 mm Hg in systolic blood pressure was found and even less of a decrement for diatolic pressure. These authors concluded that "dietary sodium restriction for older hypertensive individuals might be considered, but the evidence in the normotensive population does not support current recommendations (i.e., Dietary Guidelines Advisory Committee, 1995) for universal dietary sodium restriction". Of pertinence is the fact that the Food and Drug Administration established the daily reference value for sodium at 2400 mg (6 g of salt or 104 mmol of sodium). This is an exceedingly generous quantity of sodium when viewed from the fact that unacculturated peoples survive and thrive on amounts approximating 230 mg or less daily of the ion. Although lower than the average daily sodium intake of American adults of 3900 mg, these recommendations can be considered to be well within the hedonic range!

It would appear to be accepted by many investigators that approximately 20 percent of individuals are sensitive to modest levels of salt intake and destined to become hypertensive unless their salt intake is greatly limited (Boegehold, 1989; Sullivan, 1988; Weinberger, 1986). The favorable response of many, but not the majority of hypertensive subjects, to natriuretic drugs is evidence for a contribution of salt intake to maintenance of hypertension in salt-sensitive individuals. The myriad of other causative factors of nutritional and endogenous origin appear to participate in variable proportions among hypertensive individuals (Lenfant, 1996). The complexity of these interactions, the possibility of as yet unidentified additional factors, and the diversity of interpretation of their importance have been the subject of extensive studies and reviews (Stamler, 1993; Kannel, 1996).

It is obvious that the daily intake of sodium chloride far exceeds nutritional requirements in the majority of industrialized populations. Such satiation is difficult to avoid. Major contributing factors acting synergistically are: (1) the innate hedonic salt appetitie, (2) the wide use of sodium salts for the preservation of food and for enhancement of a salty flavor, and (3) the generally held myth by nearly all populations that an intake of mineral salt is a necessity for life. For perhaps the majority of the population, the need-free addiction to salt is no health problem. For some, it possibly is a significant agent in the pathogenesis and perpetuation of disease.

In summary, evolutionary adaptations for maintaining sodium homeostasis in environments containing a paucity of that ion are evident in all vertebrate species. The adequacy of an instinctive behavior in selection of a nutritionally balanced diet for all essential components, including sodium, has been described for two quite different human populations. Newly weaned, breast-fed infants innately selected a balanced diet over many months with resultant fully adequate growth and development. In a parallel manner, the native diets of four unacculturated groups living in no-salt societies were associated with nutritional adequacy by all measured parameters, including reproductive success. Rare examples of appetitive behavior to correct sodium deficiencies of congenital or acquired disease states document the potential strength of this instinctive drive in man.

Need-free or hedonic salt appetite is a phenomenon almost completely restricted to the human species. In previously salt-free societies, this latent appetite is easily awakened and becomes as intense as in industrialized societies living with a life-long dietary satiation with the mineral. The role of salt, sodium chloride, in the pathogenesis of disease has been a controversial issue for well over a century. Confusion between actual salt requirement and hedonic salt appetite contributes to the problem of defining the role of salt in the pathogenesis of disease. This is especially true for essential hypertension. One feasible perspective is the consideration that human salt appetite is universal, or nearly so, but the physiological responses to recognize and eliminate excesses of salt is a genetic trait which is unevenly distributed among individuals. Elucidation requires further study.

TABLE X-1: VARIETIES OF FOOD OF UNACCULTURATED PEOPLES*

	Aborigines of Australia	Yanomamö Amerindians	Bushmen of South Africa	Highlanders New Guinea
I. Animals				
A. Amphibia:	Frogs	Frogs	Frogs	Frogs; Tadpoles Toads
B. Birds	Birds Birds' Eggs	Birds Birds' Eggs	Birds Birds' Eggs	Birds Birds' Eggs
C. Fish	Crayfish Crabs Fish Mollusks	Fish Freshwater Shrimp		Eels
D. Insects	Honey Ant Larvae of Insects Moths	Catepillars Larvae of Insects Spiders	Ants and Ant Eggs Beetles Locusts Scorpions Termites	Beetles Grasshoppers Larvae of Insects Spiders
E. Mammals	Animal Bones and Marrow Bandicoots Kangaroos Opossums Wallabies Wild Dogs	Anteaters Armadillos Capybara Deer Human Bones Monkeys Peccaries Rodents Tapir	Ant Bears Anteaters Antelopes Bone Marrow Dusker Hare Lynx Porcupines Stembuck	Cassowary Cuscus Humans* Opossums Pig Rats Kangaroo Wallaby (*Previously)
F. Reptiles	Alligators Lizards Snakes Turtles/Eggs	Alligators Snakes Turtles/Eggs	Lizards Snakes Tortoises	Snakes

TABLE X-1: VARIETIES OF FOOD OF UNACCULTURATED PEOPLES*(CONT'D)

	Aborigines of Australia	Yanomamö Amerindians	Bushmen of South Africa	Highlanders of New Guinea
II. Plants				
A. Wild and Cultivated Vegetables	Various Tubers	Maize Palm Hearts Plantains Various Tubers	Beans Cucumbers Melons Various Tubers	Beans Kumu Maize Palm Hearts Plantains Sugar Cane Various Tubers
B. Flowers	Various Flowers			
C. Fruits	Various Fruits	Various Fruits	Various Fruits	Various Fruits
D. Fungi	Edible Fungi	Edible Fungi		Edible Fungi
E. Honey	Honey and Honey Comb	Honey and Honey Comb	Honey and Honey Comb	Honey and Honey Comb
F. Leaves and Stems	Various Leaves and Stems	Various Leaves and Stems		Various Leaves and Stems
G. Nuts and Seed Pods	Various Nuts and Pods	Various Nuts and Pods	Various Nuts and Pods	Various Nuts and Pods
H. Roots	Various Roots	Various Roots	VariousRoot	Various Roots

*Sources: Abbie, 1960; Basedow, 1932; Bronte-Stewart, 1960; Campbell, 1939; Chagnon, 1968; Elphinstone, 1971; Hetzel, 1978; Irvine, 1957; Jelliffe, 1962; Macfarlane, 1978; Meggitt, 1957; Oliver, 1975; Oomen, 1961; Reid, 1969; Shapera, 1960; Sorenson, 1969; Thomson, 1939.

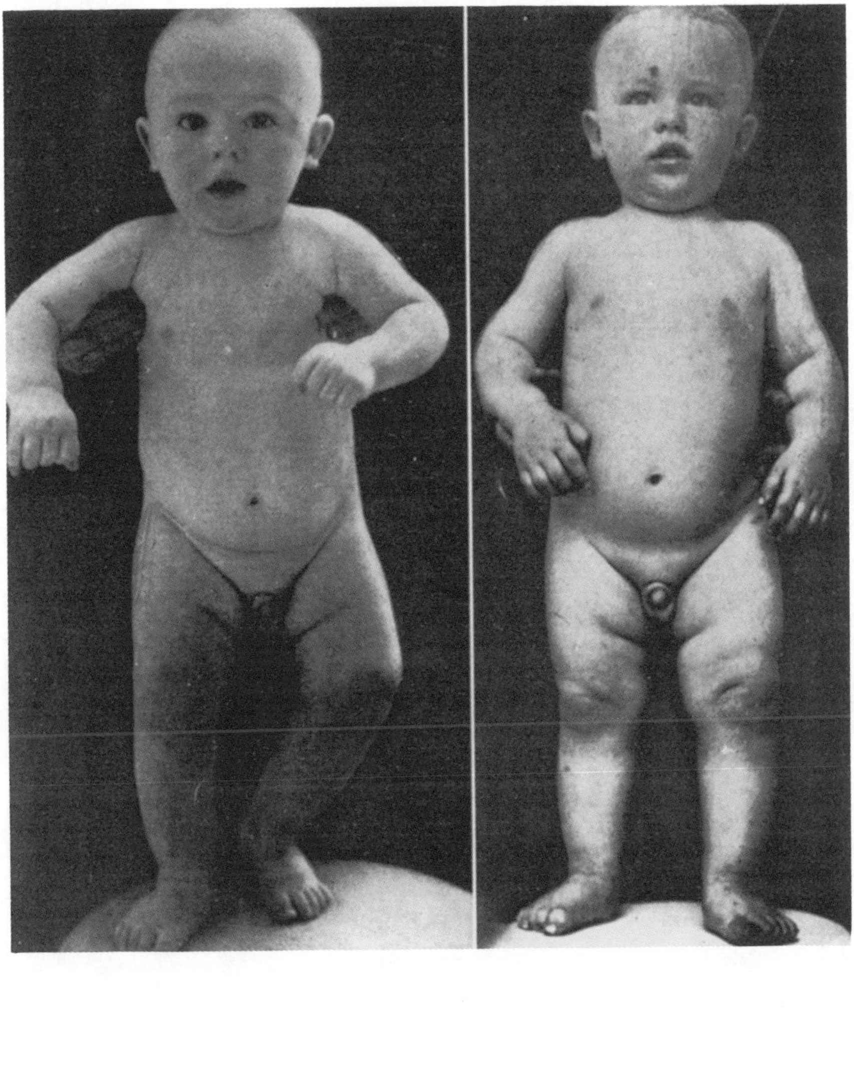

Figure X-1: Appearance of two infants following 6 and 12 months of self-selection of diet respectively. From Davis (1928) with permission.

XI. Conclusion

It has been the intent of this book to collate available reports and studies of no-salt cultures that have existed in various sites throughout the world. For a balanced presentation, the salt-using primitive societies also have been described. An appreciation of the wide distribution of the no-salt societies, the available data upon their health and the evidence of documented population expansion of several groups provide credence to a lack of nutritional disability imposed by their dietary habits.

A near-universal trait of these peoples has been the perceived primitive state of their material culture. Yet each group possessed the knowledge and physical accoutrements to survive in their environment and in many documented instances to sustain impressive population expansion. The postulated ancient routes of migration of the predecessors of native inhabitants of the several continents of North and South America, Australia and some islands of Oceania preclude consistent sources of salt or salty substances. Instead, the phylogenetically-derived mechanisms for sodium homeostatis successfully prevailed during the peopling of these areas. Another common deonominator is the virtual isolation of these cultures from industrialized contacts until the post-Columbian periods.

The existence of salt-using primitive cultures in the pre-Columbian period living in relatively close geographic proximity to the non-users adds another dimension. The origin of salt use among primitive groups can be only a speculation. The desire to obtain a salty taste is widely represented among societies first contacted in the post-Columbian period. Yet, as noted by Page (1979), proximity to the sea was not consistently associated with a high salt intake. Among individuals and among groups, hedonic salt appetite varies greatly. The extremely high daily salt intake (greater than 400 mEq/day) by Japanese of the Akita Prefecture (Sasaki, 1964) contrasts with the still generous intake (50-85 mEq/day) of some native groups including several living adjacent to the sea. Is it possible that some genetically similar people inherit a similar threshold at which salt appetite is satiated? Or, as described by Yeung (Gonzalez, 1983), parental preference is a major influence on salt appetite of their children. A parallel similar trend may exist among homogeneous populations.

The data and observations which have been presented offer no resolution to the controversy of the contribution of dietary salt in the pathogenesis of disease in contemporary societies. It is hoped that the material gives a perspective for consideration of new concepts and approaches in deciphering the roles of salt appetite and dietary salt in health and disease in industrialized societies.

Conclusion

REFERENCES

CHAPTER I:

Alpers, M and Gajdusek, DC (1965): Changing patterns of Kuru: Epidemiological changes in the period of increasing contact of the Fore people with western civilization. Am J Trop Med Hyg 14: 852-879.

Chagnon, N (1980): Personal communication.

Benton,W (1973): Salt. Encyclopaedia Britannica. Encyclopaedia Britannica, Inc, Chicago, pp. 954-955.

Dahl, LK (1958): Salt intake and salt need. N Engl J Med 258:1152-1157; 1205-1208.

Dawber, TR, Kannel, WB, Kagan, A, et al (1967): Environmental factors in hypertension. In: Stamler, J and Stamler, J (eds). *The Epidemiology of Hypertension: Proceedings of an International Symposium.* Grune & Stratton, New York. pp. 46-54.

Hartman, LF (1963): Encyclopedic dictionary of the bible. McGraw-Hill, Inc, New York, pp. 2099-2102.

Helm, J (1979): Personal communication.

Holmberg, AR (1950): *The Nomads of the Longbow: The Siriono of Eastern Bolivia.* American Museum Science Books, The Natural History Press, Garden City, New York.

Kroeber, AL (1941-42): Culture element distribution: XV. Salt, dogs, tobacco. Anthropol Rec 6:1-6.

Meneely, GR and Dahl, LK (1961): Electrolytes in hypertension: The effects of sodium chloride. Med Clin North Am 45:271-283.

Morse, WR and Bah, WT (1937): Blood pressure amongst aboriginal ethnic groups of Szechwan Province, West China. Lancet 1:966-967.

Nance, J (1975): *The Gentle Tasaday.* Harcourt, Brace and Jovanovich, New York,

Oliver, WJ, Cohen, EL, and Neel, JV (1975): Blood pressure, sodium intake and sodium related hormones in the Yanomamö Indians, a "no-salt" culture. Circulation 52:146-151.

Oliver, WJ, Neel, JV, Grekin, RJ, et al (1981): Hormonal adaptation to the stresses imposed upon sodium balance by pregnancy and lactation in the Yanomamö Indians, a culture without salt. Circulation 63:110-116.

Pickering, G (1981): Position paper: dietary sodium and human hypertension. In: Laragh, JH, Buhler, FR, and Seldin, DW (eds). *Frontiers in Hypertension Research*, reprint 1980, pp. 37-42.

Stefansson, V (1922): *My Life with the Eskimo.* The Macmillan Company, New York.

CHAPTER II:

Baxter, JP (1906): *A Memoir of Jacques Cartier: His Voyages to the St. Lawrence: A Bibliography and a Facsimile of the Manuscript of 1534 with Annotations, Etc.* Dodd, Mead and Company, New York. pp. 164-169.

References

Baxter, JP (1906): The Voyage of John Francis De La Rocque, Knight, Lord of Roberval. In: *A Memoir of Jacques Cartier: His Voyages to the St. Lawrence: A Bibliography and a Facsimile of the Manuscript of 1534 with Annotations, Etc.* Dodd, Mead and Company, New York. pp. 240-241.

Bolton, HE (1914): *Athanase De Mezieres and the Louisiana-Texas Frontier 1768-1780.* Vol 1 & 2. The Arthur H Clark Company, Cleveland.

Eskew, GL (1948): *Salt: The Fifth Element.* J G Ferguson and Associates, Chicago.

Hall, CF (1865): *Artic Researches and Life Among the Esquimaux.* Harper and Brothers Publishing, New York.

Hawkins, B (1848): *A Sketch of the Creek Country in the Years 1798-99.* Collection of the Georgia Historical Society III, Part 1. Bartlett and Welford, New York.

Helm, J (1972): The Dogrib Indians. In: Bicchieri, MG: *Hunters and Gatherers Today.* Holt, Rinehart and Winston, New York. pp.51-72.

Helm, J (1979): Personal communication.

Humfreville, JL (1899): *Twenty Years Among Our Hostile Indians.* Hunter and Company, New York.

Jouvency, J (1896): Concerning the country and manners of the Canadians, or the savages of New France. In: Thwaites, RG (ed): *The Jesuit Relations and Allied Documents: Travels and Expeditions of the French Jesuit Missionaries Among the Indians of Canada and the Northern and North-western*

States of the United States, 1610-1791. Vol 1. The Burrows Brothers Company, Cleveland.

Kroeber, AL (1941-42): Culture element distributions: XV. Salt, dogs, tobacco.Anthropol Rec 6:1-6.

de Milford, LL (1956): *Memoir or a Cursory Glance at My Different Travels & My Sojourn in the Creek Nation.* de Courcy, G (Trans), McDermott, JF (ed), R R Donnelley & Sons Company, Chicago.

Oliver, WJ, Cohen, EL and Neel, JV (1975): Blood pressure, sodium intake, and sodium related hormones in the Yanamamö Indians, a "no-salt" culture. Circulation 52: 146-151.

Oliver, WJ (1981): Unpublished data.

Quaife, MM [ed] (1917): *The Indian Captivity of O. M. Spencer.* R R Donnelley & Sons Company, Chicago.

Quaife, MM [ed] (1947: *The Western Country in the 17th Century: The Memoirs of Lamothe Cadillac and Pierre Liette.* R R Donnelley and Sons, Chicago.

Rabinowitch, IM (1936): Clinical and other observations on Canadian Eskimos in the Eastern Artic. Can Med Assoc J 34: 487-501.

Rabinowitch, IM and Smith, FC (1937): Metabolic studies of Eskimos in the Canadian Eastern Artic. J Nutr 12: 337-356.

Schoolcraft, HR (1852): *Information Respecting the History, Condition and Prospects of the Indian Tribes of the United States: Collected and Prepared Under the Direction of the Bureau of Indian Affairs.* Lippincott, Grambo and Company, Philadelphia.

References

Stefansson, V (1922): *My Life with the Eskimo*. The Macmillan Company, New York.

Swanton, JR (1918-19): An early account of the Choctaw Indians. Amer Anthropol Assoc Memoirs 22: 57-58.

Terrell, JU (1971): *American Indian Almanac*. The World Publishing Company, New York.

CHAPTER III:

August, JT, Nelson, DH, and Thorn, GW (1958): Response of normal subjects to large amounts of aldosterone. J Clin Invest 37: 1549-1555.

Barelare, B, Jr and Richter, CP (1938): Increased sodium chloride appetite in pregnant rats. Am J Physiol 121: 185-188.

Black, FL (1980): Modern isolated pre-agricultural populations as a source of information on prehistoric epidemic patterns. In: Stanley, NF and Joske, RA (eds), *Changing Disease Patterns and Human Behavior*. Academic Press (London) Ltd. pp. 37-54.

Black, FL (1981): Personal communication.

Carvalho, JJM, Baruzzi, RG, Howard, PF, et al (1989): Blood pressure in four remote populations in the INTERSALT study. Hypertension 14: 238-246.

Chagnon, NA (1968): *Yanomamö: The Fierce People*. Holt, Rinehart and Winston, New York.

Chagnon, NA (1974): *Studying the Yanamamö*. Holt, Rinehart and Winston. New York.

Chagnon, NA (1974): *Studying the Yanamamö.* Holt, Rinehart and Winston. New York.

Chagnon, NA and Hames, RB (1979): Protein deficiency and tribal warfare in Amazonia: New data. Science 203: 910-913.

Chagnon, NA (1980): Personal communication.

Chagnon, NA (1988): Life histories, blood revenge, and warfare in a tribal population. Science 239: 985-992.

Clastres, P (1972): The Guayaki. In: Bicchieri, MG (ed): *Hunters and Gatherers Today*. Holt, Rinehart and Winston. New York. pp.138-174.

Conn, JW (1949): Electrolyte composition of sweat: Clinical implications as an indication of adrenocortical function. Arch Intern Med 83: 416-428.

Córdova-Rios, M and Lamb, FB (1971): *Wizard of the Upper Amazon.*
Atheneum, New York.

Dahl, LK (1958): Sodium intake of the American male: Implications on the etiology of essential hypertension. Am J Clin Nutr 6: 1-7.

Denton, DA and Nelson, JF (1974): Effects of pregnancy and lactation on the mineral appetites of wild rabbits (*Oryctolagus cuniculus* [L]). Endocrinology 88: 31-40.

Eveland, WC, Oliver, WJ, and Neel, JV (1971): Characteristics of *Escherichia coli* serotypes in the Yanamamö, a primitive Indian tribe of South America. Infection and Immunity 4: 753-756.

References

Good, KR (1987): Limiting factors in Amazonian ecology. In: Harris, M and Ross, EB (eds): *Food and Evolution: Toward a Theory of Human Food Habits.* Temple University Press, Philadelphia. pp.407-421.

Gray, MJ and Plentl, AA (1954): The variations of the sodium space and the total exchangeable sodium during pregnancy. J Clin Invest 33: 347-353.

Hames, RB (1980): Personal communication.

Holmberg, AR (1950): *The Nomads of the Long Bow: The Siriono of Eastern Bolivia* . American Museum Science Books, The Natural History Press, Garden City, New York.

Joossens, JV, Willems, J, Claessens, J et al (1971): Sodium and hypertension. In: Fidanzo, F, Keys, A, Ricci, G et al (eds): *Nutrition and Cardiovascular Diseases,* Morgagni Edizioni Scientifiche, Rome. pp. 91-110.

Katayama, S and Yamoji, T (1982): A binding-protein for aldosterone in human plasma. J Steroid Biochem 16: 185-192.

Larrick, JW, Yost, JA, Kaplan, J et al (1979): Patterns of health and disease among the Waorani Indians of eastern Ecuador. Med Anthropol 3: 147-189.

Larrick, JW (1982): Personal communication.

Lawrence, DN, Neel, JV, Abadie, SH et al (1980): Epidemiologic studies among Amerindian populations of Amazônia. III. Intestinal parasitoses in newly contacted and acculturating villages. Am J Trop Med Hyg 29: 530-537.

Lowenstein, FW (1961): Blood pressure in relation to age and sex in the tropics and subtropics: A review of the literature and an investigation in two tribes of Brazil Indians. Lancet 1: 389-392.

Lozano, P (1873-1874): *Historia de la Conquista del l'araguay, Rio de la Plata y Tucuman Vol 1*, Buenos-Aires. pp. 412-421.

Macfarlane, WV, Skinner,SL, Scoggins, B (1970): Functional acculturation of Melanesians: I. Salts, hormones and blood pressure changes. In: Abstracts of the 42nd Congress of the Australian and New Zealand Association for Advancement of Science.

MacGillivnay, I and Buchanan, TJ (1958): Total exchangeable sodium and potassium in non-pregnant women and in normal and pre-eclamptic pregnancy. Lancet 2: 1090-1093.

McKee, HS (1955): Salt supply problems in Papua & New Guinea. S Pacific Q Bull 5: 25-26.

Meneely, GR and Dahl, Lk (1961): Electrolytes in hypertension: The effects of sodium chloride: the evidence from animal and human studies. Med Clin North Am 45: 271-283.

Mitchell, AR (1976): Skeletal sodium: A missing element in hypertension and salt excretion. Perspect Biol Med 20: 37-43.

National Research Council (1974): Recommended Dietary Allowances. (National Academy of Sciences), Edition 8, Washington, D.C.

Neel, JV, Centerwall, WR, Chagnon, NA et al (1970): Notes on the effect of measles and measles vaccine in a virgin-soil population of South American Indians. Am J Epidemiol 91: 418-429.

References

Neel, JV, Arends, T, Brewer, C et al (1972): Studies on the Yanamamö Indians. In: Human Genetics. Proc. IV Int Congr. Hum. Genet., Paris, Amsterdam: Excerpta Medica, pp. 96-111.

Neel, JV and Weiss, KM (1975): The genetic structure of a tribal population, the Yanamamö Indians: XII. Biodemographic studies. Am J Phys Anthropol 42: 25-52.

Neel, JV (1978): The population structure of an Amerindian tribe, the Yanamamö. Am Rev Genet 12: 365-413.

Nowczynski, W, Genest, J, Kuchel, O et al (1977): Age and posture-related changes in plasma protein binding and metabolism of aldosterone in essential and secondary hypertension. J Lab Clin Med 90: 475-489.

Nowaczynski, W, Landais, P, Murakami, T et al (1978a): Genetic aspects of plasma aldosterone binding globulins in families of patients with essential hypertension , including isolation of novel thermostable homologues from plasma and urine. J Steroid Biochem 11: 1027-1037.

Nowaczynski, W, Murakami, T, Richardson, K et al (1978b): Increased aldosterone plama protein binding in women on combined oral contraceptives throughout the menstrual cycle. J Clin Endocrinol Metab 47: 193-199.

Nowaczynski, W, Oliver, WJ and Neel, JV (1985): Serum aldosterone and protein-binding variables in Yanamamö Indians: A 'no-salt' culture as compared to partially acculturated Guaymi Indians. Clin Physiol Biochem 3: 289-306.

Oliver, WJ and Watson, DF (1964): Effect of salt intake on sweat electrolyes in children. Am J Dis Child 107: 470-475.

Oliver, WJ, Cohen, EL and Neel, JV (1975): Blood pressure, sodium intake, and sodium related hormones in the Yanamamö Indians, a "no-salt" culture. Circulation 52: 146-151.

Oliver, WJ, Neel, JV, Grekin, RJ et al (1981): Hormonal adaptaton to the stresses imposed upon sodium balance by pregnancy and lactation in the Yanamamö Indians, a culture without salt. Circulation 63: 110-116.

Ooman, HAPC (1961): The nutrition situation in western New Guinea. Trop Geogr Med 13: 321-335.

Raye, JR (1977): Feeding the normal newborn. In: Schaeffer, AJ and Avery, ME (eds), *Diseases of the Newborn, 4th edition,* WB Saunders, Philadelphia. pp. 840-841.

Schomburgk, R (1840-1844): *Travels in British Guiana: 1840-1844*. Translated by Roth, WE (1920). Daily Chronical Press, Georgetown, pp. 125-127.

Skinner, SL, Lumbers, ER and Symods, EM (1972): Analysis of changes in the renin-angiotensin system during pregnancy. Clin Sci 42: 479-488.

Spielman, RS, Migliazza, EC, Neel, JV et al (1979): The evolutionary relationships of two populations: A study of the Guaymi and the Yanamamö. Curr Anthropol 20: 377-388.

Tanis, RJ, Neel, JV, Dovey, H et al (1973): The genetic structure of a tribal population, the Yanomamö Indians. IX. Gene frequencies for 18 serum protein and erythrocyte enzyme systems in the Yanamamö and five neighboring tribes; nine new variants. Am J Hum Genet 25: 655-676.

References

Tapia, HR, Johnson, CE and Strong, CG (1972): Renin-angiotensin systaem in normal and in hypertensive disease of pregnancy. Lancet 2: 847-850.

United States Department of Agriculture (1975): *Handbook of the Nutritional Contents of Foods*, Dover Publications, Inc., New York.

Venning, EH and Dryenfurth, I (1956): Aldosterone excretion in pregnancy. J Clin Endocrinol Metab 16: 426-428.

Watanabe, M, Meeker, CI, Gray, MJ et al (1963): Secretion rate of aldosterone in normal pregnancy. J Clin Invest 42: 1619-1631.

Weinberger, MH, Kramer, NJ, Peterson, LP et al (1976): Sequential changes in the renin-angiotensin-aldosterone systems and plasma progesterone concentration in normal and abnormal human pregnancy. In: Lindheimer, MD, Katz, AI and Zuspan, FP (eds), *International Symposium on Hypertension in Pregnancy.* John Wiley and Sons, New York. pp. 263-279.

Weir, RJ, Pantin, DBkk, Brown, JJ et al (1971): A serial study in pregnancy of the plasma concentrations of renin, corticosteroids, electrolytes and proteins and of haematocrit and plasma volume. J Obstet Gynaecol Br Commonw 78: 590-602.

Weir, RJ, Doig, A, Frazer, R et al (1976): Studies of the renin-angiotensin-aldosterone system, cortisol, DOC, and ADH in normal and hypertensive pregnancy. In: Lindheimer, MD, Katz, AI and Zuspan, FP (eds), *International Symposium on Hypertension in Pregnancy.* John Wiley and Sons, New York, pp. 251-261.

CHAPTER IV:

Adam, JM and Ladell, WSS (1955): Report on field studies on troops of the Commonwealth Division in Korea, winter 1951-2 (Restricted). London Scientific Advisor to Army Council, cited by: Ladell, Wss and Kenny, RA, Q J Exp Physiol 40: 283-296.

Alpers, M and Gadjusek, DC (1965): Changing patterns of Kuru: Epidemiological changes in the period of increasing contact of the Fore people with western civilization. Am J Trop Med Hyg 14: 852-879.

Bellwood, PS (1980): The peopling of the Pacific. Sci Am 243:174-185.

Best, E (1902): Food products of Tuhoe land: Being notes on the food supplies of a non-agricultural tribe of the natives of New Zealand; together with some account of various customs, superstititions, etc. pertaining to foods. Trans N Z Institute 35:45-111.

Best, E (1925): *The Children of the Mist.* Vol. I, Thomas Avery and Sons, Ltd, New Plymouth.

Best, E (1952): *The Maori as He Was.* Owen, RE (ed), Government Printers, Wellington.

Brace, CL and Hinton RJ (1981): Oceanic tooth size variation as a reflection of biological and cultural mixing. Curr Anthropol 22:549-569.

Brunner, T (1851): Journal of an expedition to explore the interior of the middle island of New Zealand. J R Geogr Soc 19:344-378.

References

Choufoer, JC, van Rhijn, M, Kassenaar, AAH, et al (1963): Endemic goiter in western New Guinea: Iodine metabolism in goitrous and nongoitrous subjects. J Clin Endocrinol Metab 23:1203-1217.

Consolazio, CF, Johnson, RE and Marec, E (1951): *Metabolic Methods - Clinical Procedures in the Study of Metabolic Functions.* CV Mosby Co, St. Louis.

Craig, EWG (1964): *Man of the Mist: A Biography of Elsdon Best.* AH and AW Reed, Wellington.

Dansey, HD (1947): *How the Maoris Came to Aotearoa.* AH and AW Reed, Wellington.

Denton, DA, Nelson, JF, Orchard, E, et al (1969): The role of adrenocortical hormone secretion in salt appetite. In: *Olfaction and Taste.* Pfaffmann, C (ed), Rockefeller University Press, New York, pp. 535-547.

Dornstreich, MD and Morren, GEB (1974): Does New Guinea cannibalism have nutritional value? Hum Ecol 2:1-12.

Harsant, F (1979): *They Called Me Te Maari.* Whitcoulls Publishers, Christchurch.

Hipsley, EH and Kirk, NE (1965): Studies of the dietary intake and expenditure of energy by New Guineans. South Pacific Commission, Noumea, New Caledonia.

Inder S (1977): Pacific Islands. In: *The World Book Encyclopedia.* Vol. 15, Field Enterprises Education Corp, Chicago, pp. 6-12.

Macfarlane, WV and Skinner, SL (1970): Functional acculturation of Melanesians: I. Salts, hormones and blood pressure changes. Abstracts of the 42nd Congress of the Australian and New Zealand Association for Advancement of Science.

Macpherson, RK (1949): Tropical fatigue. University of Queensland Papers Vol. 1, No. 10, Queensland, Australia.

Maddocks, I (1967): Blood pressures in Melanesians. Med J Aust 1:1123-1126.

McKee, HS (1955): Salt supply problems in Papua and New Guinea. S Pacific Q Bull 5:25-26.

Oliver, WJ, Cohen, EL and Neel, JV (1975): Blood pressure, sodium intake and sodium related hormones in the Yanomamö Indians, a "no-salt" culture. Circulation 52:146-151.

Oomen, HAPC (1961): The nutrition situation in western New Guinea. Trop Geogr Med 13:321-335.

Oomen, HAPC (1967): Nitrogen compounds and electrolytes in the urine of New Guinean sweet potato eaters: A study of normal values. Trop Geogr Med 19:31-47.

Page, LB, Damon, A and Moellering, RC, Jr (1974): Antecedents of cardiovascular disease in six Solomon Islands societies. Circulation 49:1132-1146.

Page, LB, Moellering, RC, Jr, Lubin, N, et al (1979): Blood pressure, sodium intake and plasma renin activity in two isolated Pacific Island populations. In: *Essential Hypertension*. Thurm, RH (ed), Symposia Specialists, Inc, Chicago, pp. 11-19.

References

Prior, IAM, Evans JG, Harvey, HPB, et al (1968): Sodium intake and blood pressure in two Polynesian populations. N Engl J Med 279:515-520.

Prior, IAM, Hooper, A, Huntsman, JW, et al (1980): The Tokelau Island migrant study. In: *Population Structure and Human Variation*. Harrison, GA (ed), Cambridge University Press, Cambridge, pp. 165-186.

Reed, AW (1948): *Reed's Concise Maori Dictionary*. AH and AW Reed, Wellington.

Salisbury, RF (1962): *From Stone to Steel - Ecomomic Consequences of a Technological change in New Guinea*. Melbourne University Press, Melbourne, Australia.

Scoggins, BA, Macfarlane, WV and Skinner, SL (1980): Personal communication.

Simmons, BR (1976): *The Great New Zealand Myth*. AH and AW Reed, WellingtonSimmons, DR (1976): The great New Zealand myth: A study of the discovery in origin traditions of the Maori. Reed, H and Reed, AW (eds), Wellington.

Simmons, RT (1966): The blood group genetics of Easter Islanders (Pascuense), and other Polynesians. In: Heyerdahl, T and Ferdon, E, Jr (eds):*Reports of the Norwegian Archaeological Expedition to Easter Island and the East Pacific*, Vol. II: Miscellaneous papers, Report No. 15, Stockholm. pp. 333-343.

Sinnett, PF and Whyte, HM (1973): Epidemiological studies in a total highland population, Tukisenta, New Guinea: Cardiovascular disease and relevant clinical, electrocardiographic, radiological and biochemical findings. J Chronic Dis 26:265-290.

Sorenson, ER (1973): Mbotgate. In: Grosvenor, MB (ed): *Primitive Worlds.* National Geographic Society, Washington DC, pp. 33-56.

Sorenson, ER and Gajdusek, DC (1969): Nutrition in the Kuru region: I. Gardening, food handling, and diet of the Fore people. Acta Trop Separatum 26:281-345.

Wheatcroft, W (1973): Tifalmin: Realms of ritual - key to a world - in New Guinea. In: Breeden, RL (ed): *Primitive Worlds: People Lost in tTme.* National Geographic Society, Washington, DC, pp. 56-83.

Wheatcroft, W (1974): Personal communication.

Whyte, HM (1958): Body fat and blood pressure of natives of New Guinea: Reflections on essential hypertension. Australasian Ann Med 7:36-46.

Wills, PA (1958): Salt consumption by natives of the territory of Papua and New Guinea. Philippine J Science 87:169-177.

CHAPTER V:

Abbie, AA (1960): Physical changes in Australian Aborigines consequent upon European contact. Oceania 31:140-144.

Brace, CL (1980): Australian tooth-size Clines and the death of a stereotype. Curr Anthropol 21:141-164.

Campbell, TD (1939): Food, food values and food habits of the Australian Aborigines in relation to their dental conditions. Aust Dent J 43:1-15, 45-55, 73-87, 141-156, 177-198.

Clark, G (1969): *World Prehistory: A New Outline.* Cambridge University Press, London, 2nd edition, pp. 247-261.

References

Curtain, CC, van Loghem, E, Fudenberg, HH, et al (1972): Distribution of the imunoglobin markers at the IgCl, IgG2, IgG3, IgA2, and k-chain loci in Australian Aborigines: Comparison with New Guinea populations. Am J Hum Genet 24:145-155

Elkin, AP (1964): *The Australian Aborigines.* The Natural History Library and Anchor Books, Double Day and Co, Inc, Garden City, New York, pp. 1-25.

Flanagan, RJ (1853-54): *The Aborigines of Australia.* Sydney Empire, Sidney, pp. 59-61.

Irvine, FR (1957): Wild and emergency foods of Australian and Tasmanian Aborigines. Oceania 28:114-142.

Kirk, RL. (1977): Human Biology. In: *The Australian Encyclopedia.* Grolier Society of Australia, Sydney, pp. 16-21.

Long, JPM (1971): Arid region Aborigines: The Pintubi. In: Mulvaney, DJ and Golson, J (eds): *Aboriginal Man and Environment in Australia.* Australian National University Press, Canberra, pp. 262-270.

McArthur, M (1960): Food consumption and dietary levels of groups of Aborigines living on naturally occurring foods. In: Mountford, CP (ed), *Records of the American-Australian Scientific Expedition to Arnhem Land.* Vol 2. University Press, Melbourne, pp. 90-135.

Macfarlane, WV (1963): Endocrine functions in hot environments. In: *Environmental Physiology and Psychology in Arid Regions.* Reviews of Research, UNESCO, Paris.

Macfarlane, WV and Skinner, SL (1970): Functional acculturation of Melanesians: I. Salts, hormones and blood pressure changes. Abstracts of the 42nd Congress of the Australian and New Zealand Advancement of Science.

Macfarlane, WV (1973): Functions of Aboriginal nomads during summer. In: Kirk, RL (ed): *The Human Biology of Aborigines in Cape York.* Australian Institute of Aboriginal Studies, Canberra, pp. 49-65.

Macfarlane, WV (1978): Aboriginal desert hunters/gatherers in transition. In: Hetzel, BS and Frith, HJ (eds):*The Nutrition of Aborigines in Relation to the Ecosystem of Central Australia..* Commonwealth Scientific and Industrial Research Organization, Melbourne, pp. 49-62.

McCarthy, FD (1977): Domestic and economic life. In: *The Australian Encyclopedia.* Grolier Society of Australia, Sydney, pp. 43-49.

Meggitt, MJ (1957): Notes on the vegetable foods of the Walbiri of central Australia. Oceania 28:143-145.

Peterson, N (1978): The traditional pattern of subsistence to 1975. In: Hetzel, BS and Frith, HJ (eds): *The Nutrition of Aborigines in Relation to the Ecosystem of Central Australia..* Commonwealth Scientific and Industrial Research Organization, Melbourne, pp. 25-35.

Thompson, DF (1939): The seasonal factor in human culture, illustrated from the life of a contemporary nomadic group. In: Clark, JGD (ed): *Proceedings of the Prehistoric Society for 1939 (July - Dec).* HK Lewis and Co. Ltd., London, New Series Vol. V, part 2, pp. 209-221.

Wright, RVS (1977): Prehistory and archaeology of the Australian Aborigine. In: *The Australian Encyclopedia.* Grolier Society of Australia, Sydney, pp. 4-9.

CHAPTER VI:

Bloch, MR (1963): The social influence of salt. Sci Am 209:89-98.

Dornan, SS (1925): *Pygmies & Bushmen of the Kalahari.* Seeley, Service & Co. Limited, London, pp. 114-121.

Fourie, L (1928): The bushmen of South West Africa. In: Smit, HP (ed): *The Native Tribes of South West Africa.* Cape Times Limited, Cape Town, pp. 80-105.

Lupton, K (1979): *Mungo Park the African Traveler.* Oxford University Press, Oxford, pp. 1-10.

Maingard, JF (1937): Some notes on health and disease among the bushmen of the Southern Kalahari. Bantu Studies 11:285-295.

Park, M (1883): *The Life and Travels of Mungo Park.* R Worthington, New York.

Schweitzer, A (1939): *African Notebook,* Russel, CEB (trans), Henry Holt and Company, New York.

Shapera, I (1930): *The Khoisan Peoples of South Africa: Bushmen and Hottentots.* Routledge & Kegan Paul Ltd, London.

Truswell, AS, Kennelly, BM, Hansen, JDL, et al (1972): Blood pressures of !Kung bushmen in Northern Botswana. Am Heart J 84:5-12.

Vedder, H (1928): The Berg Damara. In: Smit, HP (ed): *The Native Tribes of South West Africa.* Cape Times Limited, Cape Town, pp. 38-61.

Wehmeyer, AS, Lee, RB and Whiting, M. (1969): The nutrient composition and dietary importance of some vegetable foods eaten by the !Kung bushmen. S Afr Med J 43:1529-1530.

CHAPTER VII:

MacLeish, K (1972): The Tasadays: Stone Age Cavemen of Mindanao. National Geographic. 142: 218-249.

MacLeish, K (1974): Personal communication.

Nance, J (1975): *The Gentle Tasaday: A Stone Age People in the Philippine Rain Forest.* Harcourt, Brace and Jovanovich, New York.

CHAPTER VIII:

Bloch, MR (1963): The social influence of salt. Sci Am 209:89-98.

Bolton, HE (1914): *Athanase de Mezieres and the Louisiana-Texas Frontier 1768-1780.* Vol. II, Arthur H Clark Company, Cleveland, pp. 187-197.

Jimenes de la Espade, M (1965): Relaciones geograficas de Indias - Peru. In: Martinez-Carreras, JU (ed), *Biblioteca de Autores Espanoles Desde la Formacion del LenguajeHasta Neustros Dias (continuacion) I and II.* Atlas, Madrid.

Kroeber, AL (1941): Culture element distributions: XV. Salt, dogs, tobacco. Anthropol Rec 6:1-6.

McArthur, M (1960): Food consumption and dietary levels of groups of Aborigines living on naturally occurring foods.

In: Mountford, CP (ed), *Records of the American-Australian Scientific Expedition to Arnhem Land.* Vol 2:90-135, University Press , Melbourne, pp. 90-135.

McKee, HS (1955): Salt supply problems in Papua and New Guinea. Pacific Q Bull 5:25-26.

Page, LB, Damon, A and Moellering, RC, Jr (1974): Antecedents of cardiovascular disease in six Solomon Islands societies. Circulaion 49:1132-1146.

Stefansson, V (1922): *My Life with the Eskimo.* The Macmillan Company, New York.

Swanton, JR (1911): Indian tribes of the lower Mississippi Valley and adjacent coast of the Gulf of Mexico. Smithsonian Institution Bureau of American Ethnology Bulletin 43, Government Printing Office, Washington, pp. 259-317.

CHAPTER IX:

Chagnon, NA (1980): Personal communication.

Hawkins, B (1848): *A Sketch of the Creek Country in the Years 1798-99.* Collection of the Georgia Historical Society III, Part 1. Bartlett and Welford, New York.

Helm, J (1979): Personal communication.

Holmberg, AR (1950): *The Nomads of the Long Bow: The Siriono of Eastern Bolivia.* American Museum Science Books, The National History Press, Garden City, New York.

Jimenes de la Espade, M (1965): Relaciones geograficas de Indias - Peru. In: Martinez-Carreras, JU (ed), *Biblioteca de*

Autores Espanoles Desde la Formacion del LenguajeHasta Neustros Dias (continuacion) I and II. Atlas, Madrid.

Kroeber, AL (1941): Culture element distributions: XV. Salt, dogs, tobacco. Anthropol Rec 6:1-6.

Macfarlane, WV, Scoggins, BA and Skinner, SL (1980): Personal communication regarding unpublished data per permission of Scoggins, BA.

Macfarlane, WV and Skinner, SL (1970): Functional acculturation on Melanesians: I. Salt, hormones and blood pressure changes. Abstracts of the 42nd Congress of the Australian and New Zealand Association for Advancement of Science.

McArthur, M (1960): Food consumption and dietary levels of groups of Aborigines living on naturally occurring foods. In: Mountford, CP (ed), *Records of the American-Australian Scientific Expedition to Arnhem Land.* Vol 2:90-135, University Press , Melbourne, pp. 90-135.

McKee, HS (1955): Salt supply problems in Papua and New Guinea. S Pacific Q Bull 5:25-26.

Page, LB, Damon, A and Moellering, RC, Jr (1974): Antecedents of cardiovascular disease in six Solomon Island societies. Circulation 49:1132-1146.

Prior, IAM, Hooper, A, Huntsman, JW, et al (1980): The Tokelau Island study. In: Harrison, GA (ed), *Population Structure and Human Variation.* Cambridge University Press, Cambridge, pp. 165-186.

References

CHAPTER X:

Abbie, AA (1960): Physical changes in Australian Aborigines consequent upon European contact. Oceania 31: 140-144.

Abraham, SF, Blaine, EH, Blair-West, JR et al (1973): New factors in control of aldosterone secretion. In: Scow, RO (ed), *Proceedings, IV International Congress of Endocrinology. International Conference Series 273*, Excerpta Medica, Amsterdam, pp. 733-739.

Abraham, SF, Blaine, EH, Denton, DA et al (1975): Phylogenetic emergence of salt taste and appetite. In: Denton, DA and Coghlan, JP (eds), *Olfaction and Taste, No. V.*, Academic Press, New York, pp. 253-260.

Barnwell, GM, Dollahite, J. and Mitchell, DS (1986): Salt taste preference in baboons. Physiol Behav 37(2): 279-284.

Basedow, H (1932): Diseases of the Australian aborigines. J Trop Med Hyg 35: 177-185; 193-198; 208-213; 229-239; 247-250; 273-278.

Benton, W (1973): Salt. Encyclopaedia Britannica. Encyclopaedia Britannica, Inc, Chicago, pp. 954-955.

Billington, BP (1960): The health and nutritional status of the aborigines. In: Mountford, CP (ed), *Records of the American-Australian Scientific Expedition to Arnhem Land.* Melbourne University Press, Parkville N.2. Victoria. 2: 27-54.

Black, D (1933): (ed), *Fossil Man in China: The Choukoutien Deposits With a Synopsis of Our Present Knowledge of the Late Cenozoic in China.* Geological Survey of China, Geological Memoirs, Series A, 11.

Blair-West, JR, Bott, E, Boyd, GW et al (1965): General biological aspects of salivary secretion in ruminants. In: Dougherty, RW (ed), *Physiology of Digestion in the Ruminant.* Butterworths, Washington, D.C., pp.198-220.

Bloch, MR (1963): The social influence of salt. Sci Am 209: 89-98.

Boegehold, MA and Kotchen, TA (1989): Relative contributions of dietary Na^+ and Cl^- to salt-sensitive hypertension. Hypertension 14: 589-583.

Bronte-Stewart, B, Budtz-Olsen, OE, Hickley, JM et al (1960): The health and nutritional status of the Kung Bushmen of South West Africa. S Afr J Lab Clin Med 6: 187-216.

Bunge, G von (1901): *Lehrbuch de Physiologie.* Vogel, Leipzig.

Busse, CD (1977): Chimpanzee predation as a possible factor in the evolution of red colobus monkey social organization. Evolution 31: 907-911.

Campbell, TD (1939): Food, food values and food habits of the Australian aborigines in relation to their dental conditions, Part I. Aust J Dent 43: 1-15.

Campbell, TD (1939): Food, food values and food habits of the Australian aborigines in relation to their dental conditions, Part II. Aust J Dent 43: 45-55.

Casley-Smith, JR (1958): The haematology of the Central Australian aborigine: I. Haemoglobin and erythrocytes. Aust J Exp Biol Med Si 36: 23-38.

Chagnon, NA (1968): *Yanomamö: The Fierce People.* Colt, Rinehart and Winston, New York.

References

Chagnon, NA and Hames, RB (1979): Protein deficiency and tribal warfare in Amazonia: New data.Science 203: 910-913.

Chagnon, NA (1980): Personal communication.

Chauncey, HH, Wallace, S, and Alman, JE (1980): Salivary chloride levels, taste threshold for salt, and food ingestion. In: Kare, MR, Fregly, NJ and Bernard, RA (eds), *Biological and Behavioral Aspects of Salt Intake*. Academic Press, New York, pp. 113-125.

Cohen, MN (1987): The significance of long-term changes in human diet and food economy. In: Harris, M and Ross, EB (eds), *Food and Evolution: Toward a Theory of Human Food Habits*, Temple University Press, Philadelphia, pp. 261-283.

Dahl, LK)1968): Salt intake and salt need. N Engl J Med 258: 1152-1157, 1205-1208.

Davis, CM (1928): Self-selection of diet by newly weaned infants. Am J Dis Child 36: 651-679.

Davis, CM (1939): Results of the self-selection of diets by young children. Can Med Assoc J 41: 257-261.

Delson, E (1992): Classification and evolutionary relationships. In: Jones, S, Martin R, and Pilbeam, D (eds), *The Cambridge Encyclopedia of Human Evolution*, Cambridge University Press, Cambridge, pp. 217-222.

Denton, DA (1957): The study of sheep with permanent unilateral parotid fistulae. Q J Exp Physiol 42: 72-95.

Denton, DA (1965): Evolutionary aspects of the emergence of aldosterone secretion in the salt appetite. Physiol Rev 45: 245-295.

Denton, DA, Nelson, JF, Orchard, E et al (1969): The role of adrenocortical hormone secretion of salt appetite. In: Pfaffman, C (ed), *Olfaction and Taste: Proceedings Third International Symposium,* Rockefeller University Press, New York, pp. 535-547

Denton, DA and Nelson, JF (1971): Effects of pregnancy and lactation on the mineral appetites of wild rabbits (*Oryctolagus Cuniculus* [L]). Endocrinology 88: 29-38.

Denton, DA (1972): Instincts, appetites and medicine. Aust NZ J Med 2: 203-212.

Denton, DA (1973a): The brain and sodium homeostasis. Conditional Reflex 8: 125-146.

Denton, DA (1973b): Sodium and hypertension. In: Sambhi,MP (ed), *Mechanisms of Hypertension, Proceedings of an International Workshop Conference, Los Angeles, 7-9 March, 1973* , Excerpta Medica, Amsterdam, pp. 46-54.

Denton, DA and Nelson, JF (1980): The influence of reproductive processes on salt appetite. In: Kare, MR, Fregly, NJ and Bernard, RA (eds), *Biological and Behavioral Aspects of Salt Intake*, Academic Press, New York, pp. 229-246.

Denton, DA (1982): *The Hunger for Salt: An Anthropological, Physiological and Medical Analysis,* Springer-Verlag, Berlin.

Denton, DA, Eichberg, JW, Shade, R. et al (1993): Sodium appetite in response to sodium deficiency in baboons. Am J Physiol 264: R539-R543.

References

DeVore, I and Washburn, SL (1963): Baboon ecology and human evolution. In: Howell, FC and Bourlière, F (eds), *African Ecology and Human Evolution*, Aldine Publishing Company, Chicago, pp. 335-367.

Drummond, JC (1934): Biochemical studies of nutritional problems. Stanford University Publications: University Series: Medical Sciences, Vol. 3, San Francisco, pp. 89-194.

Eddy, NB, Halbach, H, Isbell, H et al (1970): Drug dependence: Its significance and characteristics. In: Blachly, PH (ed): *Drug Abuse. Data and Debate (Appendix A)*, Charles C Thomas, Springfield, pp. 259-282.

Elliott, P, Stamler, J, Nichols, R et al (1996): Intersalt revisited: further analyses of 24 hour sodium excretion and blood pressure within and across populations. BMJ 312: 1249-1253.

Elphinstone, JJ (1971): The health of Australian aborigines with no previous association with Europeans. Med J Aust 2: 293-301.

Federal Register (1991): Food labeling: health claims and label statements; sodium / hypertension. 56: 60825-60855.

Fomon, SJ, Thomas, LN, and Filer, LJ, Jr. (1970): Acceptance of unsalted strained food by normal infants. J Pediatr 76: 242-246.

Fourie, L (1928): The bushmen of southwest Africa. In: Smit HP (ed), *The Native Tribes of Southwest Africa.* Capetimes Limited, Cape Town, pp. 80-105.

Fregly, NJ (1980): On the spontaneous intake of NaCl solution by dogs. In: Kare, MR, Fregly, NJ and Bernard, RA (eds),

Biological and Behavioral Aspects of Salt Intake. Academic Press, New York, pp. 55-68.

Frings, H and Frings, M (1959): Observations on salt balance and behavior of Laysen and Black-footed albatrosses in captivity. Condor 61: 304-314.

Ghiglieri, M.P. (1984): *The Chimpanzees of Kibale Forest, A Field Study of Ecology and Social Structure,* Columbia University Press, New York, pp. 72-73.

Gonzales, ER (1983): Study indicates salt is an acquired taste (editorial). JAMA 249: 2999-3003.

Good, KR (1987): Limiting factors in Amazonian ecology. In: Harris, M and Ross, EB (eds), *Food and Evolution: Toward a Theory of Human Food Habits.* Temple University Press, Philadelphia, pp.407-421.

Goodall, J (1971): *The Shadow of Man.* Houghton Mifflin Company, Boston.

Gore, R. (1997): The Dawn of Humans. National Geographic 191: No. 2: 72-99; No. 5: 84-109.

Harding, RSO (1981): An order of omnivores: nonhuman primate diets in the wild. In: Harding, RSO and Teleki, G (eds): *Omnivorous Primates: Gathering and Hunting in Human Evolution,* Columbia University Press, New York, pp. 191-214.

Hawkins, B (1848): *A Sketch of the Creek Country in the Years 1798-99.* Collection of the Georgia Historical Society III, Part 1, Bartlett and Welford, New York.

Helm, J (1979): Personal communication.

References

Henkin, RI and Soloman, DH (1962): Salt taste threshold in adrenal insufficiency in man. J Clin Endocrinol Metab 22: 856-858.

Henkin, RI, Gill, JR and Bartter, FC (1963): Studies on taste thresholds in normal man and in patients with adrenal cortical insufficiency, the role of adrenal cortical steriods and of serum sodium concentration. J Clin Invest 42: 727-735.

Hetzel, BS (1978): The changing nutrition of aborigines in the exosystem of Central Australia. In: Hetzel, BS and Frith, HJ (eds), *The Nutrition of Aborigines in Relation to the Ecosystem of Central Australia.*, Commonwealth Scientific and Industrial Research Organization, Melbourne, pp. 39-47.

Hladik, C.M. and Gueguen, D.J. (1974): Géographie et nutrition minérale chez les primates sauvages. Cr Acad Sci, Paris 279 D, 1393-1396.

Hladik, C.M. (1977): Chimpanzees of Gabon and chimpanzees of Gombe: some comparative data on diet. In: Clutten-Brock, T. H. (ed), *Primate Ecology: Studies of Feeding and Ranging Behavior in Lemurs, Monkeys and Apes*, Academic Press, London, pp. 481-501.

Hodges, KJ, Fysh, CF, and Rienits, KG (1950): The New Guinea and Papuan food composition tables. In: Hipsley, EM and Clements, WF (Eds): Report of the New Guinea Nutrition Survey Expedition1947, Part 9. Commonwealth Department of Health for the Department of External Territories. Government Printer. Sydney.

Hodges, KJ (1960): Report of the biochemical assessments of nutritional status. In: Mountford, CP (ed), *Records of the American-Australian Scientific Expedition to Arnhem Land.* Melbourne University Press, Parkville N.2. Victoria. 2: 27-54.

Holmberg, AR (1950): *The Nomads of the Longbow: the Siriono of Eastern Bolivia,* American Museum Science Books, The Natural History Press, Garden City, New York, pp. 1-104.

Howard, R (1850) *A Treatise on Salt, Showing Its Hurtful Effects on the Body and Mind on Man, and on Animals, Especially CONSUMPTION, as Taught by the Ancient Egyptian Priests and Wise Men in Accordance with the Author's Experience, 2nd Edition.* W and T Piper, London. pp. 12-46.

Idler, DR, Ronald, AP, and Schmidt, PJ (1959): Isolation of cortisone and cortisol from the plasma of specific salmon (*Onchorynchus Nerka*). J Med Chem Soc 81: 1260.

Intersalt Cooperative Research Group (1988): Intersalt: an international study of electrolyte excretion and blood pressure. Results for 24 hour urinary sodium and potassium excretion. BMJ 297: 319-328.

Irvine, FR)1957): Wild and emergency foods of Australian and Tasmanian aborigines. Oceania 28: 114-142.

Itani, J and Nishimur, A (1973): The study of infrahuman culture in Japan: A review. In: Montagna, M (ed), *Symposium Fourth International Congress of Primatology,* Vol 1, Karger, Basel, Switzerland, pp. 26-50.

Jelliffe, DB, Woodborn, MA, Bennetat, FJ, et al (1962): The children of the Hoadza hunters. J Pediatr 60: 907-913.

Kannel, WB (1996): Blood pressure as a cardiovascular risk factor: prevention and treatment. JAMA 275: 1571-1576.

Kaunitz, H (1956): Causes and consequences of salt consumption. Nature 178: 1141-1144.

References

Kawai, M (1965): Newly acquired pre-cultural behavior of the natural troop of Japanese monkeys on the Koshima islet. Primate 6: 1-30.

Kawamura, S (1954): A new type of action expressed in feeding behavior of Japanese monkeys in the wild. Seibutsu Shinka 2: (1).

Kelley, J (1992):Classification and evolutionary relationships. In: Jones, S, Martin R, and Pilbeam, D (eds), *The Cambridge Encyclopedia of Human Evolution*, Cambridge University Press, Cambridge, pp. 223-230.

Langley, D (1950): Food consumption and dietary levels. In: Hipsley, EM and Clements, WF (Eds):Report of the New Guinea Nutrition Survey Expedition1947, Part 4. Commonwealth Department of Health for the Department of External Territories. Government Printer, Sydney.

Lawick-Goodall, J Van (1968): The behavior of free-living chimpanzees in the Gombe Stream Reserve. In: (eds), Cullen, JM and Beer, CG) *Animal Behavior Monographs* 1: 161-311.

Leakey, MG, Feibel, CS, McDougall, I et al (1995): New four-million-year-old hominid species from Kanapoi and Allia Bay, Kenya. Nature 376:
565-571.

Leakey, RE and Lewin, R (1977): *Origins.*, EP Dutton, New York.

Lehmann CG (1883): *Lehrbuch der Physiologischen Chemie, 2nd Edition,* Engelmann, Leipzig.

Lenfant, C (1996): High blood pressure: some answers, new questions, continuing challenges (Editorial). JAMA 275: 1604-1606.

Macfarlane, WV (1978): Aboriginal desert hunter/gatherers in transition. In: Hetzel, BS and Frith, HJ (eds), *The Nutrition of Aborigines in Relation to the Ecosystem of Central Australia.*, Commonwealth Scientific and Industrial Research Organization, Melbourne, pp. 49-62.

Manley, JJ (1884): Salt and other condiments. In: Gamgee, A (ed): *Physiology of digestion and the digestive organs, The Health Exhibition Literature, Vol. 4,* Health in Diet, International Health Exhibtion, William Clowes and Sons, Ltd, London, pp. 641-784.

McArthur, M (1960): Food consumption and dietary levels of groups of aborigines living on natural occurring foods. In: Mountford, CP (ed), *Records of the American-Australian Scientific Expedition to Arnhem Land,* Melbourne University Press, Parkville N 2. Victoria. 90-135.

McKee, HS (1955): Salt supply problems in Papua and New Guinea. South Pacific Quarterly Bulletin 5: 25-26.

Martin, R (1992): Classification and evolutionary relationships. In: Jones, S, Martin R, and Pilbeam, D (eds), *The Cambridge Encyclopedia of Human Evolution*, Cambridge University Press, Cambridge, pp. 17-23.

Medical Research Council (1948): Vitamin C requirement of human adults: A preliminary report by the Vitamin C Subcommittee of the Accessory Food Factor Committee, Lancet 1: 853-858.

Meggitt, MJ (1957): Notes on the vegetable foods of the Walbiri of Central Australia. Oceania 28: 143-145.

References

Midgley, JP, Matthew, AG, Greenwood, CMT et al (1996): Effect of reduced dietary sodium on blood pressure: A meta-analysis of randomized controlled trials. JAMA 275: 1590- 1597.

Morris, JG and Gartner, RJW (1971): The sodium requirements of growing steers given an all-sorghum grain ration. Br J Nutr 25: 191-205.

National Research Council [U.S.A] (1948): Recommended Daily Allowances.Reprint and Circular Series, No. 129, Sec. 2. Washington, D.C. p. 23.

National Research Council. Subcommittee on Dairy Cattle Nutrition (1978): Nutrient Requirements of Dairy Cattle, Nutrient Requirements of Domestic Animals, No 3, Fifth Revised Edition, National Academy of Sciences, Washington, D.C.

Neel, JV, Arends, T, Brewer, C et al (1972): Studies on the Yanomamö Indians. In: Human Genetics, Proceedings Fourth International Congress of Human Genetics, Paris, Amsterdam. Excerpta Medica, pp. 96-111.

Neel, JV (1994): *Physician to the Gene Pool: Genetic Lessons and Other Stories.* John Wiley and Sons, New York, p. 150.

Nishimura, H (1980): Comparatiave endocrinology of renin and angiotensin. Adv Exp Med Biol 130: 29-77.

O'Brien, D and Chase, HP (1979): The assessment of nutrition status in individuals and population group. In: Barness, L (ed), Pediatric Nutgrtion Handbook, American Academy of Pediatrics, Evanston, Illinois, pp. 7-90.

Oliver, WJ and Watson, DF (1964): Effect of salt intake on sweat electrolytes in children. Am J Dis Child 107: 470-475.

Oliver, WJ (1972): Personal observations.

Oliver, WJ, Cohen, EL, and Neel, JV (1975): Blood pressure, sodium intake, and sodium related hormones in the Yanomamö Indians, a "no-salt" culture. Circulation 52: 146-151.

Oliver, WJ (1976): Personal observations.

Oliver, WJ, Neel, JV, Grekin , RJ, et al (1981): Hormonal adaptation to the stresses imposed upon sodium balance by pregnancy and lactaton in the Yanomamö Indians, a culture without salt. Circulation. 63: 110-116.

Oliver, WJ (1987): Personal observations.

Oomen, HAPC (1961): The nutrition situation in western New Guinea. Trop Geogr Med 13: 321-335.

Pangborn, RN (1967: Some aspects of chemoreception in human nutrition. In: Kare, MR and Maller, O (eds), *Chemical Sensors and Nutrition,* Johns Hopkins Press, Baltimore, pp. 45-60.

Peterson, N (1978): The traditional pattern of subsistence to 1975. In: Hetzel, BS and Frith, HJ (eds), *The Nutrition of Aborigines in Relation to the Ecosystem of Central Australia.*, Commonwealth Scientific and Industrial Research Organization, Melbourne, pp. 25-35.

Philips, JG, Holmes, WN, and Bondy, PK (1959): Adrenal corticosteroids in salmon plasma (*Onchorynchus Nerka*). Endocrinology 65: 811-818.

Platt, BS (1950): Tables of representative values of foods commonly used in tropical countries. Medical Research Council Special Report Series No. 253, Reprinted 1950. His Majesty's Stationary Office, London.

References

Ramsay, DJ and Reid, IA (1979): Salt appetite in dogs. Fed Proc 38: 3906.

Reid, LH and Gajdusek, DC (1969): Nutrition in the Kuru region: II. A nutritional evaluation of traditional Fore diet in Moke Village in 1957. Acta Trop. Separatum 26, No. 4: 331-345.

Remkema, JA, Senshu, T, Gaillard, BDE et al (1962): Regulation of sodium excretion and retention by the intestine in cows. Nature 195: 389-390.

Richter, CP (1943): Total self-regulatory functions in animals and human beings. Harvey Lectures 38, Science Press Printing company, Lancaster, Pennsylvania, pp. 63-103.

Richter CP and Mosier, HD, Jr. (1954): Maximum sodium chloride intake and thirst in domesticated and wild Norway rats. Am J Phyhsiol 176: 213-222.

Roberts, W (1897): Digestion and diets. Second Edition, London

Robizon, B, Kare, MR, and Beauchamp, GK (1980): Comparative aspects of salt preference and intake in birds. In: Kare, MR, Fregly, NJ and Bernard, RA (eds), *Biological and Behavioral Aspects of Salt intake*, Academic Press, New York, pp. 69-81.

Rosenberger, AL (1992): Classification and evolutionary relationships. In: Jones, S, Martin R, and Pilbeam, D (eds), *The Cambridge Encyclopedia of Human Evolution*, Cambridge University Press, Cambridge, pp. 208-216.

Schaller, GB (1963): *The Mountain Gorilla: Ecology and Behavior.*, University of Chicago Press, Chicago, pp. 149-169.

Schapera, I (1930): *The Khoisan Peoples of South Africa: Bushmen and Hottentots*. Routledge & Kegan Paul, Ltd, London, pp. 91-101.

Schleiden, MJ (1875): Das Salz. Leipzig.

Schomburgk, R (1922): Travels in British Guiana: 1840-1844. Roth, WE (Trans), Daily Chronicle Press, Georgetown, pp. 125-127.

Scoggins, BA, Blair-West, JR, Coghlan, JP et al (1970): Physiological morphological response of mammals to changes in their sodium status. *Memoirs Society Endocrinology No 18, Symposium: Hormones and the Environment,* Cambridge University Press, London, pp. 577-602.

Sillen, A and Brain, CK (1990): Old flame: burned bones provide evidence of an early human use of fire. Natural History 99: 6-10.

Simons, E (1992): Classification and evolutionary relationships. In: Jones, S, Martin R, and Pilbeam, D (eds), *The Cambridge Encyclopedia of Human Evolution*, Cambridge University Press, Cambridge, pp. 199-208.

Smith, SE and Aines, PD (1959): Salt requirements of dairy cows. Cornell Agric Exp Stn Bull No 938.

Sorenson, ER and Gajdusek, DC (1969): Nutrition in the Kuru region: I. Gardening, food handling and diet of the Fore people. Acta Trop. Separatum 26, No. 4: 280-330.

Stahl, A, (1984): Hominid diet before fire. Current Anthropology 25:
151-168.

Stamler, J, Stamler, R, Neaton, JD (1993): Blood pressure, systolic and diastolic, and cardiovascular risks: US population data. Arch Intern Med. 153: 598-615.

References

Stringer, CB (1992):Classification and evolutionary relationships. In: Jones, S, Martin R, and Pilbeam, D (eds), *The Cambridge Encyclopedia of Human Evolution,* Cambridge University Press, Cambridge, pp. 241-251.

Sullivan, JM, Prewitt, RL and Ratts, TE (1988): Sodium sensitivity in normotensive and borderline hypertensive humans. Am J Med Sci 295: 370-377.

Teleki, G (1981): The omnivorous diet and eclectic feeding habits of chimpanzees in Gombe National Park, Tanzania. In: Harding, RSO and Teleki, G (eds), *Omnivorous Primates: Gathering and Hunting in Human Evolution,* Columbia University Press, New York, pp. 303-661.

Telecki, G (1973): *The Predatory Behavior of Wild Chimpanzees.* Bucknell University Press, Lewisburg.

Thomson, DF (1939): The Seasonal factor in human culture, illustrated from the life of a contemporary nomadic group. In: Clark, JGD (ed), Proceedings of the Prehistoric Society (new series 5, part 2), HK Lewis and Co. Ltd, London, pp. 209-221.

Thorn, GW, Dorrance, SS, and Day, E (1942): Addison's disease: Evaluation of synthetic desoxycorticosterone acetate therapy in 158 patients. Ann Intern Med 16: 1053-1096.

US Dept of Agriculture, US Dept of HEalth and Human Services. *Nutrition and Your Health* 4th ed. Washington, DC: US dept of Health and Human Services; 1995.

Wallace, AR (1853): Travels on the Amazon. Ward Lock, London.

Weiffenbach, JM, Daniel, PA, and Cowart, BJ (1980): Saltiness in developmental perspective. In: Kare, MR, Fregly, NJ and Bernard, RA (eds), *Biological and Behavioral Aspects of Salt Intake,* Academic Press, New York, pp. 13-29.

Weinberger, MH, Miller, JH, Luft, FC et al (1986): Definitions an d characteristics of sodium sensitivity and blood pressure resistence. Hypertension 8 (suppl II): II-127--134.

Wilkins, L and Richter, CP (1940): A great craving for salt by a child with corticoadrenal insufficiency. JAMA 114: 866-868.

Wood, BA (1992): Classification and evolutionary relationships. In: Jones, S, Martin R, and Pilbeam, D (eds), *The Cambridge Encyclopedia of Human Evolution,* Cambridge University Press, Cambridge, pp. 231-240.

Wrangham, RW (1975): Behavioural ecology of chimpanzees in Gombe National Park, Tanzania. Ph.D. thesis, University of Cambridge, Cambridge.

Wrangham, RW (1977): Feeding behavior of chimpanzees in Gombe National Park, Tanzania. In: Clutten-Brock, T. H. (ed), *Primate Ecology: Studies of Feeding and Ranging Behavior in Lemurs, Monkeys and Apes,* Academic Press, London, pp.503-538.

CHAPTER XI:

Gonzalez, ER:(1983) Study indicates salt is an acquired taste. JAMA 249:2999-3000.

Page, LB, Moellering, RC, Jr., Lubin, N, et al: (1979) Blood Pressure, Sodium Intake, and Plasma Renin Activity in Two Isolated Pacific Island Populations. In: Thurm, RH (ed),

Essential Hypertension, Year Book Medical Publishers, Chicago, pp. 11-19.

Sasaki, N: (1964) The relationship of salt intake to hypertension in the Japanese. Geriatrics 19:735-744.
